POSTGRADUATE PAEDIATRICS SERIES

under the General Editorship of
JOHN APLEY
C.B.E., M.D., B.S., F.R.C.P., J.P.
Emeritus Consultant Paediatrician, United Bristol Hospitals

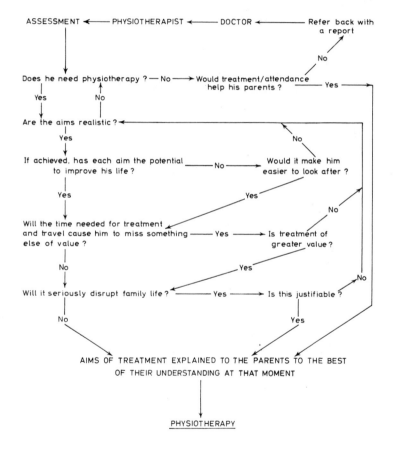

Some questions relating to out-patient treatment

Physiotherapy in Paediatric Practice

DAVID SCRUTTON M.Sc., M.C.S.P.

Superintendent Physiotherapist,
Newcomen Centre,
Guy's Hospital, London

MOYNA GILBERTSON M.C.S.P.

Group Superintendent Physiotherapist,
Department of Physical Medicine,
Hospitals for Sick Children,
Great Ormond Street, London

BUTTERWORTHS
London and Boston

THE BUTTERWORTH GROUP

ENGLAND
Butterworth & Co (Publishers) Ltd
London: 88 Kingsway, WC2B 6AB

AUSTRALIA
Butterworths Pty Ltd
Sydney: 586 Pacific Highway, NSW 2067
Melbourne: 343 Little Collins Street, 3000
Brisbane: 240 Queen Street, 4000

CANADA
Butterworth & Co (Canada) Ltd
Toronto: 2265 Midland Avenue,
Scarborough, Ontario, M1P 4S1

NEW ZEALAND
Butterworths of New Zealand Ltd
Wellington: 26–28 Waring Taylor Street, 1

SOUTH AFRICA
Butterworth & Co (South Africa) (Pty) Ltd
Durban: 152–154 Gale Street

USA
Butterworth
161 Ash Street,
Reading, Mass. 01867

First published 1975

© Butterworth & Co (Publishers) Ltd, 1975

ISBN 0 407 00017 8

Suggested UDC Number 615.8–053.2

Filmset by V. Siviter Smith & Co Ltd, Birmingham
Printed in England by Chapel River Press, Andover, Hants.

Contents

vii

Foreword

There are good reasons why practising paediatricians should, at their level, be well informed about the physiotherapy of infants and children.

Many physiotherapists have a special knowledge of children and their parents and their reactions to stresses. Paediatricians are wise to take trouble to learn from them. This we can do only if we understand their ways of thinking and the aims, scope and methods of the treatments they give and how they relate to parents. Conversely the only physiotherapist available to help the paediatrician's patient may be fresh from her basic training in which she has had little teaching about neurodevelopmental disorders and she may have no access to a more senior physiotherapist or to a specialist in physical medicine. In their co-operative action to help the child, the physiotherapist will, in such a situation, need help and the person to give it will be the doctor who knows children and who should, at his level, know about physiotherapy for them. With every child the therapy will be better if therapist and doctor with mutual understanding meet to discuss the child and pool their respective knowledge and experience for the benefit of the child and his parents.

This book is by two physiotherapists with great experience in therapy and a fresh approach in thinking about their subject. It fills a major need. It was for me most illuminating and valuable. Look, for instance, at the balanced discussion of the various schools and methods of physiotherapy on page 49. It is now much clearer to me to what degree any method of physiotherapy is to be judged on the theoretical basis put forward by its proponents. Finding out exactly what each method has to offer each child is not easy for the eclectic practitioner whether of physiotherapy, of paediatric rehabilitation or of paediatrics. If we are to help the children and to come nearer to an evaluation of the usefulness of treatments, the paediatrician needs to watch the physiotherapist at work with the child and his parent.

The authors have considered a wide variety of treatments, they have taken from many of them, and present their own practice with clarity and conviction, for doctors to read and learn. Physiotherapists will find it an extremely informative text which they will enjoy reading.

This is not a long book; sometimes it is concentrated, but for all doctors who deal with children it is highly rewarding to have read, to have at hand to consult and to read again.

Ronald Mac Keith, D.M., F.R.C.P.

Preface

The aim has been to describe paediatric physiotherapy as it is, or as it could well be. This is not a book about what might be possible in a physiotherapy orientated world, but rather what the authors consider to be a reasonable compromise between the possible in theory and the achievable in practice. Anyone can appear to treat better by doing more, but in doing so is in danger not only of placing unreasonable demands on the patient and his family but also of being able to do less for other patients.

It is hoped that this book will help the doctor decide when and how physiotherapy can help his child patients. It may also show how in some conditions the physiotherapist can increase the doctor's effectiveness, whilst simultaneously reducing the time the doctor need spend with the parent or child. The book is written primarily for doctors; but the authors, both physiotherapists, naturally hope that it will also be useful to others, particularly nurses and all those concerned with the care of handicapped children. The simple line diagrams may help as reminders as well as for teaching purposes.

Since this is not written as a treatment manual for physiotherapists, the authors have avoided the usual text-book style in favour of a discussion of physical treatment. Whilst physiotherapists may find the book unconventional, the authors hope they will not find it unstimulating.

D.S.
M.G.

Acknowledgements

Many people have helped us in many ways. The authors would particularly like to thank Dr E. D. R. Campbell for his helpful advice at the planning stage; our professional colleagues, especially Miss McTear, Mrs Reid and Miss Tipping; and Gordon Halcrow, Brunel University. We are grateful to our secretaries who have been very patient.

Most of all we thank those members of our families who have been there only, but always, when needed.

Introduction

Most people know what is meant by physiotherapy but it is not easy to define. What it is has never been fully resolved within the profession since (except for the satisfaction of the administrative mind) there seems little need to do so. Any definition of physiotherapy tends to include several other professions, all with their own distinct disciplines, such as occupational therapy, speech therapy, remedial gymnastics and chiropody. The overlap of areas of treatment is large and the physiotherapist's precise function may be determined as much by that individual's aptitudes as by the local facilities provided by the other disciplines. For instance, in the absence of an occupational therapy department the physiotherapist has to place greater emphasis on the activities of daily living, and when speech therapists are not available some of their functions may be taken by the physiotherapist.

Definition

Any concise definition of physiotherapy cannot help being too exclusive or too inclusive, for physiotherapy involves the modification of the patient's physical external environment, either generally or topically, so as to promote healing or otherwise improve the body's efficiency. Such a simple and wide definition embraces all the physical treatments and much else besides: for example, it is not considered physiotherapy to apply a hot compress to a boil, or to advise a patient to go to bed and keep warm. Moreover not all physiotherapy is physical treatment. A large part consists of advice: in paediatric physiotherapy this is usually advising adults on the day-to-day care of a child.

Professions, however, are not defined by their boundaries. It is their aims, and the concepts behind the means of achieving those

1

aims, which can tell us most. Why is there a need for physiotherapy? What needs are not already met by the other healing professions? The present situation results from the historical development of medicine which until comparatively recent times was forced, through lack of knowledge of the *milieu interieur*, to rely on therapy through the external environment—physical therapy is 'perhaps the oldest form of treatment known to man' (1). Galen divided exercises for children into three types (*a*) self-produced, (*b*) produced by someone else, and (*c*) produced by medical direction; and, not unreasonably, added that the third variety is not adapted to the healthy (2). Francis Glissen (1597–1677) recommended suspension exercises for rickets, together with 'broaths and panadaes'* (3), whilst by 1918 Kurt Huldschinsky treated this condition by artificially produced ultra-violet radiation (4). Earlier, Oscar Bernhard (b.1861) had used natural sunlight in the treatment of suppurating and indolent wounds (4). Massage has had many advocates, including Ambroise Paré (1510–1590), surgeon to four kings of France (5).

Many of these empirical methods have been retained because their validity and convenience are self-evident. Some treatments were superseded or discarded as increasing knowledge destroyed their rationale; but a large number of treatments, whose validity remained unchallenged, were gradually left out of general medical practice. There were several reasons for this, the chief being time: time to learn about the methods and to carry out the treatment— for effective physiotherapy requires both of these.

Consequently, over the past fifty to one hundred years a distinct discipline has grown up which covers a large body of therapy, apparently separate and yet complementary to medicine and surgery.

Age and treatment

Just as children's medicine is nòt at all a junior version of adult medicine, so children's physiotherapy is *quite unlike* adult physiotherapy. The use of adult treatment aims and methods can lead to much unnecessary treatment; moreover, a large number of children do just as well untreated as treated. Result? The belief in some quarters that most physiotherapy with children is a waste of time. It is not so, but if this is to be convincingly demonstrated, the basis

---

* panada=breadcrumbs boiled to a pulp in milk, broth, or water and variously flavoured (e.g. with nutmeg).

for selection of patients and the rationale of treatment must be completely different from those used for adults.

Referral

Physiotherapists have been extensively trained and are competent to examine those patients referred to them so as to select the appropriate physical treatment. They may treat only a patient who has been initially referred by a doctor and this is for their own protection as much as the patient's. It is a restriction which should be enjoyed by the physiotherapist rather than resented, since specializing in one form of treatment has automatically limited the scope of knowledge too much for the situation to be otherwise. Nevertheless, receiving patients by referral only does have serious disadvantages. Unless selection is made by someone fully conversant with physiotherapy there is always the possibility that the patients are referred too late or are not those that can be helped most. Naturally it is impossible for physiotherapists to know of the patients they do not see, but the other side of the coin is very apparent. It can be both embarrassing and frustrating to be referred a child who can *not* be helped, particularly when the parents have already been assured by someone whose opinion they respect that what their child needs is 'physiotherapy'. It is also embarrassing when a child who will get better without treatment is referred: for example, some children with 'flat feet' etc.

Communication

Mistaken referrals do occur and this is partly due to a lack of time for the medical profession to enquire further—there are many topics of more immediate importance—but it is equally because the findings, treatments and results of physiotherapy are seldom reported back to the doctor. The lack of feedback from the physiotherapist fosters mistaken referrals and does nothing to put her in touch with those whom she might have treated effectively. On occasions it seems that physiotherapy departments are used as Reception Centres for all those patients needing some form of attention but whom the doctor cannot fit neatly into other departments.

It is sometimes assumed that, since a physiotherapist's knowledge of medical conditions is limited, it is likewise limited in all fields. On the contrary we consider that with many disorders (particularly those relating to the locomotor system) the physiotherapy department can contribute fresh information and insight on the management of a patient. If it cannot, then there is something wrong with that department: and a hospital usually has the physiotherapy department it deserves. A department which has patients referred by interested people will inevitably become an invaluable asset. For the patient's and parents' sake the situation must be avoided in which the physiotherapist thinks the doctor doesn't understand while the doctor thinks that she doesn't know!

The plan of the book

As a result, in planning this book, the authors decided to divide it into two main sections. Section II is the practical part, but first let us discuss the aim of Section I. This is to give a concept of what physiotherapy is about: how the physiotherapist thinks about a patient and a disorder and how she sets about her treatment. It is divided into chapters, most of which cover an area of treatment rather than a particular disorder, because physiotherapy for children treats mainly symptoms not causes. Where specific disorders are mentioned they are usually as examples to help clarify a general picture.

It is our experience that a knowledge of medicine may make it initially more difficult to understand physiotherapy: for a physiotherapist does not always look at a patient or disease 'like a doctor only less so', but often from a different point of view. It is not easy to see an old friend as with the eyes of a stranger.

Occasionally in Section I we have prefaced the description of treatment with a passage which should not be taken out of context. We consider this to be necessary if the reader is to appreciate fully what follows.

Section II is divided into disorders. They are arranged in alphabetical order and since a detailed explanation of the physical treatment techniques could fill a small library, there is a section on 'further reading' which should satisfy the reader interested in greater detail. Section II is intended for quick reference and each disorder is dealt with under three headings: Discussion, References to Section I, and Further Reading. In brief, then, Section I is intended for reading, Section II for reference. The Appendices deal either with matters common to several chapters or with subjects inappropriate to the other sections.

Clinical trials

It has not been our aim to discuss the details of treatment (except to clarify a general principle) or the relative merits of one treatment method against another. Few treatments have been subjected to clinical trials. This statement may be surprising and needs enlarging upon. Physiotherapists tend to be untheoretical and to a small extent this is a cause for the lack of controlled trials. The main cause lies in the many difficulties which have to be overcome. These difficulties obviously vary with the condition being considered and the particular treatments, but it is hard to think of any physiotherapy treatment which allows the setting-up of a double-blind trial, since the physiotherapist cannot help but know whether she is carrying out a treatment or a placebo. Equally, most treatments will tell the patient which trial group he is in. Further, the criteria of success are often hard to define: healing of an ulcer by ultra-violet irradiation can be easily plotted (area, time and dosage), but it is difficult to measure how well someone walks—it is more than just the sum of muscle strengths, joint ranges, speed and endurance. What gait looks like may be more important than all these and can only be subjectively evaluated. To a certain extent the electrical treatments can be standardized by intensity and time, but most treatments are not so easily defined. Physiotherapy is not simply a science; in fact for some of the treatments it would be wrong to consider it a science at all. The treatment is a result of a particular attitude of mind, a way of observing a patient and considering a condition, a way which is built on a sound knowledge of anatomy, physiology, exercise theory etc., but cannot always be said to follow directly from it. There is a large element of empiricism which, in some cases, has developed into a school of thought. Although often referred to as a 'method', it is more usually a concept of how patients should be treated: a set of priorities from which a style of treatment naturally flows.

This must be appreciated by the doctor if he is to avoid the assumption that treatment by 'A's method' in one hospital is identical to treatment by the same method elsewhere. It seldom is, although the influence of the treatment attitude will be apparent and perhaps add to the confusion. This situation is not unique to physiotherapy but is very relevant to any discussion of it.

REFERENCES

(1) Stenn, F. (1967), *The Growth of Medicine*, Springfield, Ill.: Thomas.

(2) Still, G. F. (1965). *The History of Paediatrics,* p 33. London: Dawson.
(3) Ibid. (1965). citing Glissen's *Treatise on Rickets* (1650), p. 226.
(4) Krusen, F. H. (1971). *Physical Medicine.* London: W. B. Saunders.
(5) Singer, C. and Ashworth Underwood, E. (1962). *A Short History of Medicine,* p. 371. Oxford: Clarendon Press.

THE ESSENCE OF PHYSIOTHERAPY FOR CHILDREN

CHAPTER 1

How much treatment?

Once it is decided that physical treatment can probably be of help to the patient the problem becomes one of what sort of treatment and how much. For acute disorders the decision is usually straight-forward, but for chronic disorders it is not so simple. If altering the child's physical external environment in certain ways can benefit his function, it could be asserted that he should be given the maxi-mum treatment. Perhaps so, but fortunately for him his disability is not the only thing in his life, nor can he be the only consideration. He is a person, not a disease; part of a family which has its own time-consuming needs and also much to offer him in affection and in general upbringing. So, whilst the aims of treatment must be dictated primarily by the child, the means of treatment are con-trolled by his total environment.

Although early, accurate and complete diagnosis of some con-genital disorders is difficult, a child is seldom too young for treatment to be started. In some conditions (e.g. spina bifida, cerebral palsy) the importance of treatment may diminish as the child grows older, either because it seems to be less effective or because of other more important demands on his time. It may become prominent again for short periods as surgery is required. One problem in discussing the quantity of treatment is deciding where physiotherapy begins and good handling ends.

It is sometimes difficult to suspend treatment of a patient when further progress might be made. However, continuation of treatment is not solely a matter of whether he could improve with further help, but of priorities. How much of his time should be taken up acquiring what may be a small return in improved function? Some of the factors which should concern the doctor and physiotherapist are shown in the frontispiece. There can be no hard and fast rules: a compromise must be found depending on many factors:

Age of the patient

Babies, needing full-time care by their mothers, are usually readily available for treatment, although appointments must allow for their sleep/feed routine. Provided their mothers are not out at work, pre-school children are usually available for treatment. Later on school attendance may present a problem unless the child is at a special school which provides physiotherapy.

Severity and type of handicap

A greater disability does not necessarily need more treatment.

The parents' ability to co-operate

This depends on their attitude to the child, intelligence, size of their family and distance from the treatment centre.

The criteria for deciding what constitutes a continued need for treatment will vary from patient to patient: what may be an insignificant improvement in one child can be important to another. The aim should be to get the optimum overall benefit from a treatment regime and not necessarily the maximum physical result. After all, physiotherapy is but one aspect of the child's total environment. At certain times it may be the most important, at others of no importance. It must never become an end in itself, but remain one of the means by which a child is given the opportunity whereby he may lead as complete and fulfilled a life as possible.

CHAPTER 2

Parent counselling and the physiotherapist

When a child becomes an out patient at a physiotherapy department he usually brings a worried parent and is himself worried and
tense. A few parents are satisfied with the explanations they have
had and their understanding of what is wrong with their child and,
after a brief look at the treatment, are content to let it perform its
ritual magic. But most parents are not satisfied with their knowledge
of what is wrong, what is going to be done, what effect it will have,
how long it will all take and what the outcome will be. Furthermore,
they are concerned also about what their own parents or neighbours
have told them since they saw the doctor!

The doctor will have explained, but he may not have been fully
understood. Understanding takes time, discussion and repetition.
To a parent the physiotherapist is an ideal person with whom to
have a discussion because:

she is there;

she obviously understands what is wrong (she wears a uniform);

she is an 'outsider' (she wears a uniform and is not a doctor);

she is seen regularly enough for a relationship to develop;

and she is already giving the parent and child advice—for this
may be much of the outpatient treatment. Advice necessarily
leads to questions and from then on the floodgate is open.

If the therapist is faced with questions beyond the immediate
treatment should she answer them? Yes, unless there is an obvious
reason not to, or if the questions are outside her competence. She
must answer unless she is continually to appear totally ignorant and
a cypher.

The patient–physiotherapist relationship can be as important as the patient–doctor relationship and in some conditions it may be more so.

In the chronic disorders the parents usually have many deep and ill-defined worries, which only time and discussion can bring into the open. Discussion, yes: but with the physiotherapist? Why not? And who else? Who else combines the opportunity, time and knowledge? For it appears that most parents find it easier to introduce their problems when the resulting discussion is seemingly of secondary importance. The apparent prime purpose of their visit to the physiotherapy department is to learn how to handle and treat their child. Although opportunities can be deliberately created, there is no pressure to raise a particular worry. Once raised, it can be discussed in conversation or, if preferable, un-selfconsciously put aside by overt concentration on the job at hand—treating the child. With a percipient physiotherapist this allows the parents a freedom of discussion without any sense of compulsion, that is, without the feeling 'I am supposed to discuss my worries'.

Some of the problems raised by the parents or evident to the physiotherapist cannot be dealt with by the physiotherapist and are referred to the physician. He is unlikely to be immediately available but he can be advised of the problem and the parents can be given an appointment to see him in the near future. In this way the physiotherapist becomes an effective extension of the doctor as well as a filter. The large majority of worries, questions and problems are well within the scope of anyone with day-to-day experience of handling children and often problems, which would otherwise be referred to a Medical Social Worker or Health Visitor, are resolved immediately. Some of these can be answered in the form of 'idle talk' during treatment; others merit a more formal approach. If it becomes apparent that, although they accept what the physiotherapist says, they would like to hear it from their doctor, this will be arranged.

The key to this arrangement is trust. Trust by the physiotherapist in the parents' capacity to make a most valuable contribution to their child's treatment; trust by the parents that the physiotherapist knows her job; trust by the physician in the physiotherapist's experience and judgement and a reciprocal trust by the physiotherapist in her more senior colleague. Most parents want to do what is best for their child and, if they seem not to be doing so, it is less likely to be their fault than that of the professional team.

Parent associations

Many parents find that membership of the parent association concerned with their child's disorder is very helpful and they often hear of these organizations for the first time when attending the physiotherapy department.

CHAPTER 3

Respiratory disorders

1. DISCUSSION

The basic principles of chest physiotherapy are instilled into the physiotherapy student very early in her training. Patients requiring—or who have been prescribed—breathing exercises are often among the first entrusted to her care. The physiotherapist therefore has a built-in emphasis placed on chest conditions. Medical students and doctors may come in contact with physiotherapy only on the ward, and since by far the largest part of physiotherapy for *in*patients is for chest conditions, either real or imaginary, some members of the medical profession are likely to think of physiotherapists almost entirely as chest technicians. Over the years this false impression has led to the routine prescribing of breathing exercises in many acute illnesses, almost all pre- and post-operative situations and in recurrent chronic chest conditions. We think this has fostered an automatic approach on the part of the therapist with the result that she has less time (and probably expertise) for those in real need and, in turn, may promote a lack of confidence on the part of the doctor. The emergence of untrained 'inhalation therapists' in some quarters is a regrettable result of the belief that chest care is easy and physical therapy can be largely replaced by the use of inhalations and mechanical devices. Apparatus may have a useful role to play but the authors regard this general trend as retrograde.

Basically the therapist has four tools to use in the treatment of all chest conditions: postural drainage, breathing exercises, posture control and family advice. Each of these will help to improve exercise tolerance but will need to be modified to suit the particular patient: it is here that the skill lies and nowhere is this more apparent than with children.

The techniques of treatment will vary with the size of the child and more importantly with his attitude and the attitude of his parents. For example it is unusual for a child with a chronic chest condition to accept easily the need for regular treatment and much patience may be required from the whole family. Family advice takes time, but it is time well spent.

Postural drainage is especially important in any condition where there are excessive secretions or areas of lung collapse. Drainage positions depend upon the zones requiring drainage and are modified according to the immediate condition of the patient. Posture is combined with percussion or vibrations, as appropriate. In the treatment of babies and young children breathing exercises are usually performed 'passively' or are taught as games. If it is necessary to teach specific localized breathing techniques, great care must be taken to ensure that this does not make the child tense. Posture is always of great importance and the needs may range from checking the nursing position of the acutely ill to encouraging a child with a chronic chest condition to join in vigorous games and mobility exercises.

Lung disease in early childhood does not cause only direct damage to the lung tissue, but may also interfere with the development and growth of the lung structures (6). Therefore a primary aim must always be to treat children as soon as or even before (e.g. cystic fibrosis) symptoms appear, in an effort to help prevent lung damage and maintain normal tissue growth.

2. EXAMINATION BY THE PHYSIOTHERAPIST

Relevant facts needed by the therapist

From the doctor

It is essential that the therapist is given an adequately comprehensive diagnosis and informed of any factor which might modify the vigour of the treatment (e.g. a cardiac defect). It is useful to know the specific areas of collapse. Armed with such information the therapist will carry out her own examination and be able to plan treatment.

General observations

The general attitude of the child and apparent relationship with any accompanying adult must be noted. It must be remembered that first impressions often need to be modified as the therapist becomes better acquainted with the family: a child visiting an outpatient department for the first time may be entirely absorbed in proving that the unknown adults, probably in white, are being truthful when they say he is going home. Consequently, it may not be until the second visit that any treatment is possible. Nevertheless, a good initial rapport is essential and devoting the first encounter to acclimatization is never wasted. The family may need assurance that obvious antagonism from the child towards the therapist is normal. While the therapist is talking to the family and playing with the child she notes aspects of the breathing pattern and posture which may need further examination at the appropriate moment. It may appear to a doctor that the therapist is unnecessarily slow in making her first assessment, but if a child needs to attend a physiotherapy department regularly and the parents are to be helped they must positively want to come. 'Make haste slowly' is usually a good motto for the first few appointments.

Examination of breathing patterns

Visual

The examination should take place in a warm relaxed atmosphere. The therapist will first observe the type of quiet breathing pattern; the rate, depth, general area and whether accessory muscles of respiration are used. These observations will be made with a baby in lying position and for a child in half lying, then standing, and repeated following activity.

At the first assessment a note is made of the child's general posture. This is considered in more detail in 'Methods of Treatment' below.

Palpation

This may not be necessary and can be positively unhelpful, as touching the child may cause an immediate and marked change in his breathing pattern. An experienced therapist may add to her knowledge by placing her hands gently but firmly on the chest and feeling irregularities in depth of breathing in specific areas.

Auditory

It is now almost universally accepted that a therapist working in an intensive care or thoracic surgery unit should be properly instructed in the use of a stethoscope. This will help her to concentrate her treatment on those areas where secretions are collecting. We need hardly add that clinical experience is necessary to become proficient with a stethoscope and this skill can only be acquired by a therapist who has the opportunity to work as part of a medical team. For most chronic chest conditions a therapist will not need to use a stethoscope.

Exercise tolerance

It is helpful to establish a base line for the evaluation of future treatment. Simple tests can be evolved according to the age and status of the patient at the first interview to determine his level of exercise tolerance and these can be recorded at suitable intervals to assess his progress. A Vitalograph (7) or Wright peak flow meter may be used to record vital capacity. The tests carried out routinely by therapists in many paediatric hospitals are forced vital capacity and expiratory volume. Additionally, it is gradually becoming more usual for them to help in the laboratory with more sophisticated respiratory function tests.

3. METHODS OF TREATMENT

The means available are: (*a*) Postural drainage; (*b*) Breathing exercises; (*c*) Posture control; and (*d*) Family advice.

Postural drainage

We consider that for many conditions this is the most important aspect of physiotherapy. If the lungs are blocked with secretions, it would be unreasonable to expect an improvement in breathing pattern or decrease in respiratory distress until secretions are cleared. In chronic chest conditions, especially cystic fibrosis, it is a waste of time trying to improve posture or exercise tolerance until the secretions are removed or lessened. At the same time it must be emphasized that postural drainage cannot be considered in isolation and any comprehensive treatment plan will usually incorporate drainage with breathing exercises, or breathing exercises with posture control etc.

From her examination and knowledge of the anatomy of the bronchial tree the therapist can select appropriate postures (*see Figures 1-10*). Posturing of the child is often an essential part of home treatment and the child's parents will need careful instruction. Lying in one position for a length of time is very tedious for any child, and every effort is made to prevent boredom and encourage him to understand the importance of the procedure as early as possible. (*See* 'Family Advice' below.)

Postural drainage position

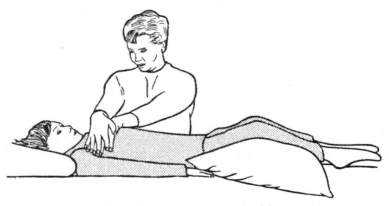

Figure 1. Anterior segment: upper lobes

Postural drainage positions

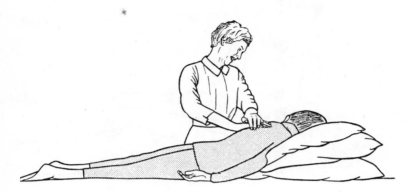

Figure 2. Posterior segment (left): upper lobe

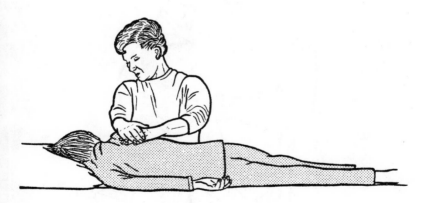

Figure 3. Posterior segment (right): upper lobe

Postural drainage positions

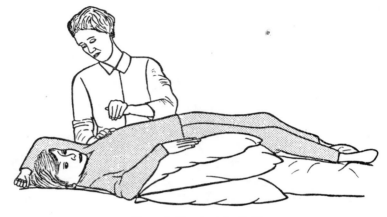

Figure 4. Lingular lobe (left)

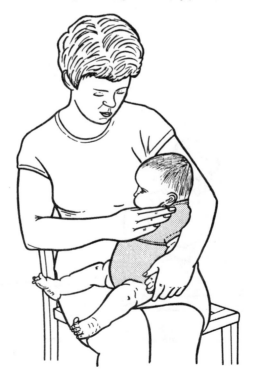

Figure 5. Apical segment: upper lobes

Postural drainage positions

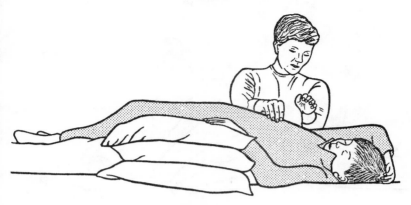

Figure 6. Middle lobe (right)

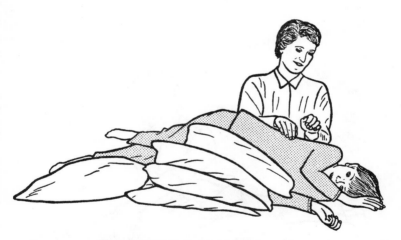

Figure 7. Lateral segment (right): lower lobe

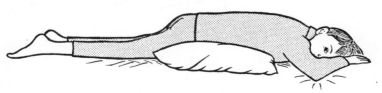

Figure 8. Apical segments: lower lobes

Postural drainage positions

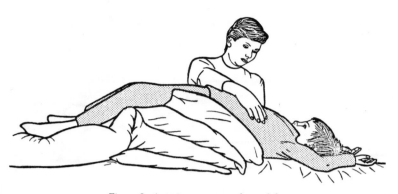

Figure 9. Anterior segments: lower lobes

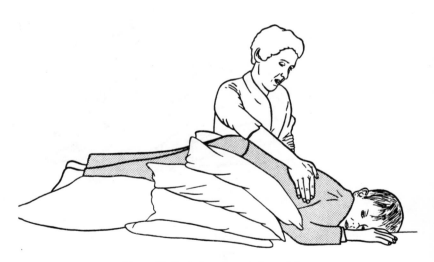

Figure 10. Posterior segment: lower lobes

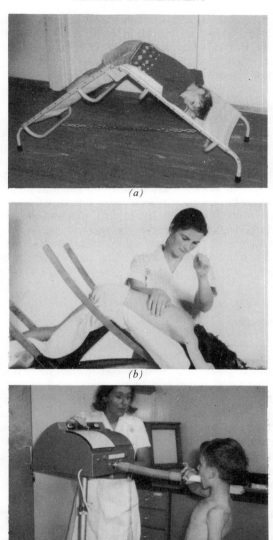

*Figure 11. (a) Basal segment, lower lobes: using a tipping frame.
(b) An equally effective tipping frame at home. (c) A child
using a Vitalograph*

Postural drainage is usually combined with percussion and vibrations. Percussion and vibration have a similar aim—to aid expectoration. For percussion a loosely cupped hand strikes the patient gently, firmly and rhythmically: this is usually known as 'clapping'. For vibrations the therapist's hands are in contact with the patient's chest, giving a shaking movement during expiration. Vibrations are used in combination with clapping and most particularly when the condition of the patient forbids more vigorous treatment. The aim is to stimulate coughing and improve as well as assist expectoration. In acute conditions vibrations are given during breathing out and the child will require frequent short treatments throughout the day and possibly the night. In chronic disorders treatment sessions are usually longer and less frequent, but it is impossible to prescribe a fixed length of time for any session. The more vigorous treatment, percussion, is usually reserved for children with productive chronic conditions, and is combined with vibrations. Once again, when home treatment is necessary, thorough instruction of the parents is of supreme importance.

Breathing exercises

Very few people use their breathing apparatus economically and this is often due to poor postural habits. However, there is so large a respiratory reserve that few problems arise, and happily in the normal course of events nobody needs to think about breathing or doing breathing exercises. Even so there are those who advocate their importance as part of everyday life, just as there are conversely those who consider breathing exercises have no part to play in the treatment of any chest condition. As is so often the case, the truth lies between these two extremes.

Relaxation is an important part of treatment. We do not consider that breathing exercises should be taught 'in through the nose and out through the mouth', or that all breathing should be performed with the mouth closed. Every child must be trained according to his own specific needs. The aims are to establish a relaxed and improved breathing pattern and the means should be within the capabilities of any therapist undertaking paediatric physiotherapy.

Teaching parents how they should teach their children is a vital and most difficult part of the therapist's task.

'Passive' breathing exercises

Many occasions arise when patients require chest care but are totally unable to co-operate, e.g. neonates, comatose or semi-comatose paralysed patients. There may be medical or surgical reasons for a child to be nursed on or off a respirator. In these situations the therapist helps to maintain a clear airway by using manual pressure; and vibrations or percussion on expiration take the place of breathing exercises. Rate and depth of respiration can be influenced in this way and expectoration aided.

Postural control

Postural control cannot be dissociated from breathing exercises. Bad posture is often the most immediately noticeable characteristic of a child with chronic chest disease. Typically there are two types of faulty posture: (a) lax droopy posture, i.e. apparent flat feet, 'kissing' knees, pot belly, poking chin, and round shoulders; (b) tense posture, i.e. knees pushed back, shoulders raised, neck tense and a rigid thorax.

Both groups benefit from treatment, but the idea that there is one correct posture must be discounted. Any adherence to the old-fashioned knees back, tummy in, shoulders back, chin in 'army' posture is to be deplored as it succeeds only in substituting one bad posture for another. Essentially a good posture should be aesthetically pleasing, relaxed, graceful and supple. For children with chronic chest conditions the greatest danger is lack of thoracic mobility, possibly combined with tenseness. If a programme of treatment starts early general mobility exercises will help to maintain relaxation, but if the patient has developed an habitual tenseness, then emphasis will need to be placed on relaxation first and afterwards on mobility. (*See* Asthma, Section II.)

A proper combination of postural drainage, breathing exercises and postural control should lead to an improved exercise tolerance, and hence to the possibility of a more normal life for the whole family.

Family advice

The constant aim must be to help children to lead their lives as normally as possible; and parents of children with chronic chest conditions will require more help from the physiotherapist than those with acute illness. Inevitably some parents will be apprehensive. They know that exposure to infection is more hazardous for their children than for others, or that they are more likely to become ill, e.g. cystic fibrosis. They will need much support and encouragement so that their children are adequately supervised and yet not molly-coddled.

It is essential that parents are thoroughly taught:

(1) What to do at home.

(2) How often to do it, having discussed when best to fit it into the day's routine.

(3) Why they are being asked to do it.

(4) To establish an informal link with the physiotherapy department so that they never feel abandoned. No matter how well the family seems to be containing the situation at home it is important that their attitude and methods are checked from time to time, at least at every routine visit to the doctor. This not only reassures the family that their treatment techniques are sound, but emphasizes the hospital's continuing interest in their problems. Various pamphlets and films have been produced as an aid to home treatment, but we think these should only be used in conjunction with advice from a therapist. A teaching film, for example, usually covers as many aspects of treatment as possible, but few points will be relevant to each family and viewing without the opportunity to discuss points raised may be self-defeating by causing confusion. Although domicillary visits are apparently time consuming, a visit by a physiotherapist well known to the family can be so helpful that in the long term time is saved.

There are several parent associations and families should be informed about these. Meeting other people with similar problems can be helpful. Many parents want, and therefore should be encouraged, to become involved in fund raising for research: (this may apply more particularly to those with very severely affected children, or children with genetically determined disease). Very occasionally we think parents are pressurized and made to feel that membership of an association is obligatory. This is undesirable, and parents who feel resistant to, or uncomfortable in, a group must have their right to abstain respected. Although they are mentioned in this section parent associations are not confined to children with chest conditions and similar worries may arise in other situations (*see* Chapter 2). Parents may feel that if they join a group they are admitting that their child has a worse disorder than they are at present willing to admit.

4. RESPIRATORY CONDITIONS

It is convenient to consider the treatment of respiratory conditions in two main groups:

(*a*) Surgical conditions: (*i*) Non-thoracic surgery
(*ii*) Thoracic surgery

(*b*) Medical conditions: (*i*) Acute
(*ii*) Recurrent
(*iii*) Chronic

SURGICAL CONDITIONS

Non-thoracic surgery (8)

Routine pre- and post-operative breathing exercises are inappropriate and obsolete for children; indeed recent studies throw doubt on their usefulness at any stage. The average baby and young child ventilates adequately by crying and is usually so mobile in bed that secretions do not stagnate. Sometimes, known 'chesty children' require pre-operative treatment and these should also be checked post-operatively.

Thoracic surgery

Aims of treatment

(*a*) To clear lungs of secretions pre- and post-operatively.
(*b*) To prevent accumulation of secretions post-operatively.
(*c*) To prevent post-operative pulmonary collapse.
(*d*) To facilitate exchange of gases in the lungs by keeping the air passages clear and so help to prevent respiratory insufficiency.
(*e*) To re-expand collapsed areas.

Pre-operative treatment (8)

This is not usually required but it is useful if the physiotherapist has met the older patient and parents to explain what may be necessary post-operatively.

Post-operative treatment

Recent changes in many operative techniques have vastly diminished the need for intensive physiotherapy, and this is no longer prescribed routinely in most hospitals. Nevertheless, there is a need for a 24-hour service to deal with those patients who do present post-operative problems. For such children treatment may start four hours after return from theatre and will consist, if their condition allows, of vibrations with the patient lying first on one side and then on the other and suction to the tracheostomy or endotracheal tube and to the nasopharynx. Treatment is governed by the current status of the patient. The frequency necessary may vary from every two hours to only once a day; it is essential for the therapist to be in close touch with the medical and nursing staff. This is one of the situations where it must be recognized that the boundaries between nursing and physiotherapy are very ill-defined. A 24-hour service is a departure from physiotherapy tradition, and owing to universal shortage of staff it is always difficult and sometimes impossible to implement. Adequate patient care can be maintained only if nurses and therapists work together.

MEDICAL CONDITIONS

Acute

Physiotherapy can contribute in the treatment of many acute medical conditions. These will range from specific chest infections which may be comparatively trivial or very grave, to conditions where, due to trauma (e.g. road traffic accident) or to a systemic disease (e.g. meningitis), there is depression of normal breathing or coughing. Intensive treatment is required for a varying length of time and the therapist will use drainage and breathing exercises as appropriate.

Recurrent

There are some long-standing medical chest conditions (e.g. asthma) in which the child may be comparatively healthy between episodes and so should not properly be included in the chronic group. When the episodes occur they will need intensive treatment, possibly including physiotherapy.

Chronic

The whole range of chest physiotherapy is brought into action in the treatment of chronic respiratory conditions. Many patients (*see* cystic fibrosis) will require physiotherapy management throughout life and parental advice is often the most important facet of the therapist's work (*see* Chapter 2).

5. APPARATUS

Mist tents

There is a wide divergence of opinion about the use of mist tents in the treatment of chest conditions. There are many attendant problems. Moreover the efficiency of droplet penetration has yet to be proven.

Possible indications for use

Clearing the chest of tenacious mucus. A moist atmosphere may help infants with high respiratory rate, who are mouth-breathing by humidifying the inspired air and so easing the removal of mucus.
Sore throat and trachea. Mist may sooth and help to reduce oedema.
Oxygen therapy. If a child requires oxygen it should be at least at ambient temperature and humidified.
Tracheostomy. A child with a tracheostomy is unable to warm and humidify inspired air in the normal way. He must therefore be helped so that the mucosa does not become dry, leading to hardening of mucus.

Difficulties

(1) Possible introduction of infection.
(2) Possible danger of overhydration.
(3) Possibility of overheating or overcooling.
(4) Production of increased secretions even though less viscous.
(5) Resistance of patient who may be uncomfortable or frightened.
(6) Rotting beds and mattresses, particularly important if home use is contemplated.

Positive pressure ventilators

These can be used to give intermittent positive pressure breathing (IPPB) using a mask or mouthpiece or tracheostomy connection. They may be used to re-educate weak respiratory muscles or when post-operative respiratory complications are evident. They are also used to administer drugs through a nebulizer. When the cough reflex is suppressed IPPB is sometimes combined with vibrations.

In general, from a physiotherapy point of view, positive pressure ventilators play only a small part in the management of children.

Air compressors

These are more commonly used to administer drugs by nebulizer, and are effectively used at home, e.g. for cystic fibrosis. The machines are easy to manage, and disposable masks have eliminated many of the cleaning problems.

Spinhaler insufflators

Used to administer some drugs, e.g. Intal, in ultra-fine powder form by oral inhalation. The dangers are well known but they are easy to use and maintain, and are of particular value in the administration of antispasmodics to alleviate or prevent attacks of asthma, as they can easily be carried about by the patient.

Tipping frames

The chests of babies can be drained by tipping over an adult's knee. Otherwise some form of aid is required. Laying children over a pile of pillows or the end of a divan may suffice, but sometimes a frame is more comfortable. The simplest variety which can be folded and stored easily at home is best. Many hospital departments have adjustable beds, plinths or very sturdy and expensive frames to perform the same task, but these are not necessary for family use (*see Figure 11b*).

Automatic percussion apparatus

A variety of mechanical aids is available. At the moment none of them seems to be entirely satisfactory. The jacket type is expensive, delicate and complicated and therefore liable to fail. They are all difficult to maintain, and less efficient than manual percussion. Since the adolescent needs to be encouraged towards independence the hope is that more refined apparatus will soon become available.

REFERENCES

(6) Reid, L. (1971). 'Lung growth, the facts.' *C.F. News*, **6**, 2 and 3.
(7) Vitalograph Ltd (1964). *Use of the Vitalograph.*
(8) Nichols, P. J. R. and Howell, D. (1974). 'Routine, pre- and post-operative physiotherapy—a preliminary trial.' *Physiotherapy*, **56** (8), 356.

CHAPTER 4

Movement disorders and orthopaedic situations

1. THE PHYSIOTHERAPIST'S EXAMINATION OF THE CHILD WITH A MOVEMENT DISORDER OR RETARDATION

This chapter outlines the features which are part of a full examination of a child with any movement disorder. The primary purpose of the examination is to find out what the child can do, what he cannot do, and the factors responsible for limiting his movement ability. The examination also gives the therapist time to orientate herself to the child and his difficulties—and the child time to do the same with the therapist. Wherever possible the parents should be present. This helps in gaining their confidence by showing that the physiotherapist is thorough and knows how to handle their child in spite of his difficulties: something the parents may not yet have achieved.

Certain points are covered, although the child's age and the movement disorder will affect their relevance. Each physiotherapist places emphasis on those parts of the examination which relate directly to her treatment.

(*a*) *Relevant facts not directly related to the movement examination*

The physiotherapist notes any facts which may affect the patient's development, his treatment, or his movement disorder. These should have been included in the referral letter. Of particular importance are impaired vision or hearing, mental subnormality, epilepsy and its current drug therapy, and anything else which is likely to influence his handling (for instance a disorder of the cardiovascular system, a Spitz–Holter valve or a hiatus hernia). The use of glasses or a hearing aid should be noted.

(b) Apparatus

Wheelchairs, calipers, below-knee irons, special boots and spinal supports are checked.

(c) Surgery

A note is made of past surgery, usually orthopaedic, which may influence movement ability.

(d) Deformity

Structural: clinically apparent or probable dislocation or sub-luxation, varus or valgus deformity of bones and limb shortening. There are two main types of shortening: (*i*) primary, which may be severely incapacitating; and (*ii*) secondary to a movement disorder. Upper limb shortening is seldom of importance to movement, although it can be inconvenient cosmetically and for clothing. The lower limb shortening is significant only if the child is likely to stand and walk, when it can have a marked effect on spinal posture and gait.

Fixed: altered range of movement caused by epithelial or connective tissue. The range of movement may vary with the position of other joints if the cause is muscle contracture.

Postural: disorders of posture, caused by unbalanced muscle action.

(e) Muscle power (9)

Strangely enough the strength of a muscle, acting as a prime mover, is not always of paramount importance to either function or treatment. There are several reasons for this:

(1) In upper motor neurone disorders testing muscles for strength has little significance: when and how the muscle functions, as well as its usual postural length, are more important.

(2) Good co-ordination of the available muscle power can produce a quality of movement out of all proportion to the apparent strength recorded on a chart.

(3) The strength of a muscle may vary at different points of its range.

(4) In myopathies and other degenerative conditions there is little that can be done to increase muscle power and so testing for strength has only overall assessment value.

However, there are situations where grading muscle power is essential and the standard method in this country is by use of the Medical Research Council 0–5 scale (10) (and *see p. 70*).

(f) *Postural and movement ability*

This varies markedly with the child's age and disability. His postural and movement ability is examined where appropriate in supine, prone, all sitting positions, on all fours, in upright kneeling, half-kneeling, standing, walk-standing and one leg standing. Any difficulties in achieving or maintaining a position, carrying out normal movements in those positions, or balance and protective responses are noted.

Movements from one position to another are observed: rolling, crawling, getting up to sitting, up to standing, walking, running, hopping, going up and down stairs etc. Depending upon the child's age and movement ability observation is then extended to activities of daily living (in the first instance by asking the parents).

Whether a movement can be carried out or a posture maintained is itself of interest, but far more important is *how* it is done.

(g) *Other information*

When relevant to treatment brief notes are made of: (i) sucking, dribbling, swallowing, chewing, speech; (ii) bowel and bladder control; (iii) any other difficulties the parents have noticed.

The aim of the examination is to build up a pattern of the patient's capacities, his difficulties, the essential problems and the likely outcome of treatment.

As in all things, experience allows some short cuts to be taken, but when this is done care is needed as it is so often the anomalies in movement ability which give the best clue to treatment. The full examination may take little time for a child who is mildly or severely handicapped; on the other hand it can take several visits to complete if he has a moderate disorder or is unable to co-operate.

The initial examination is not final; it is the first step in an assessment which continues all the time the child is being treated.

2. MOVEMENT DISORDERS

(a) CEREBRAL PALSY AND SIMILAR DISORDERS

(I) CLASSIFICATION OF CEREBRAL PALSY AND SIMILAR MOVEMENT DISORDERS

It is customary to distinguish these movement disorders in two ways by:

(1) The clinical signs (spastic, hypotonic, athetoid etc.).

(2) The distribution (quadriplegia, hemiplegia etc.).

These classifications are used by physiotherapists and give useful information about the patient, but they are diagnostic rather

TABLE 1

Classification of Cerebral Movement Disorders for Physical Treatment

	Type	Factors relevant to treatment
The primary functional disability	Difficulty in producing movement (p.36)	Hypertonia Hypotonia
	Difficulty in preventing (involuntary) movement (p.37)	(1) Type of involuntary movement (2) How it disrupts voluntary movement (3) Degree of hypertonia (4) Emotional influence
	Difficulty in controlling movement (ataxia) (p.39)	(a) Type of movement involved (b) Additional motor difficulties
The age of onset of the lesion (p.39)	(1) Congenital (2) Acquired (a) before 1 year (b) between 1 and 5 years (c) after 5 years	

than treatment categories. For the physiotherapist there are two additional and relevant methods of classification which make it easier to appreciate these disorders (Table 1).

(3) The primary functional disability.

(4) The age of onset of the lesion.

Primary functional disability

Difficulty in producing movement: This is caused either by hypertonia, hypotonia* or frequently a combination of the two (Table 2).

TABLE 2

Primary Functional Difficulty: Type 1—Difficulty in Producing Movement

Cause	Resistance to passive movement	Factors influencing the distribution of hypertonia
Hypertonia	Spastic Spastic/plastic Plastic	Mass patterns Tonic postural responses Associated movements
Intermittent hypertonia superimposed on hypotonia	Variable	
Hypotonia	Reduced None	

Hypertonia has three interrelated variables: (*a*) degree; (*b*) distribution; (*c*) character. These vary from patient to patient and within the same patient under different circumstances.

The degree of hypertonia will depend on many immediate factors, not the least of which are the competence with which the child is handled and the child's emotional state. Within this variability each child can be considered to have an average degree of hypertonia which can then be described as 'severe', 'moderate', 'mild' etc. However, this very variability is also important. Thus hypertonus in a particular child can be thought of as having both a 'mean' and a 'mean deviation'. Those children with a high mean

---

* It is considered that these terms are generally understood and that any attempt at precise definitions is out of place.

deviation are very difficult to treat as their response is so widely variable and their tonic responses appear almost phasic.

The distribution of hypertonia is constant in the sense that it is confined to certain areas of the body in a particular child, but variable in that it may shift from one muscle group to another within those areas. There are usually one or more preferred postures, which are adopted if circumstances permit and are the child's positions of rest. These postures are characteristic of the different disorders and are influenced by several factors (Appendix 2): (*a*) mass patterning of movement; (*b*) pathological and primitive tonic responses; and (*c*) associated movements.

The character of the hypertonus refers to the response to passive stretching. There are patients who have a purely spastic response, and a few who have only a plastic response, but most have a combination of the two, the spastic element being predominant.

Hypotonia. This is obviously not a precise term. There are degrees of hypotonia, for it is unlikely that a cerebral defect will produce a hypotonia which is constant in all circumstances. The term 'zero cerebral' for a flaccid muscle or muscle group is sometimes used and is appropriate if it is appreciated that it may be applicable only to a particular set of circumstances. Extreme hypotonia may persist in all circumstances but if, as the child matures, the hypotonia gives way to hypertonia, then abnormal tonic responses will also appear. For treatment purposes it is useful to imagine that these responses were present all the time, but are suppressed by lack of muscle action. Usually these tonic responses first appear as phasic alterations of posture.

Difficulty in preventing involuntary movement (*see* Table 1). Both the hypertonic and hypotonic states are comparatively easy to classify because they are fundamentally static and therefore the postures—or the lack of postures—can be described. The descriptions may not be all-embracing but they give a semblance of being so and provide a basis from which to observe. The involuntary movement disorders permit no such simple method of classification, for although there are quite distinct types of involuntary movements (and some disorders fall readily into one category or another) there are infinite shades of difference making subdivision impossible.

Phelps (11) divided cerebral palsies with involuntary movement into eleven groups which he considered relevant to his treatment methods; but in our experience, once a classification of this sort is started, the possibilities are infinite for, as Crothers and Paine (12) observed, it is partly aetiological, partly topographical and partly descriptive.

Our own classification is for use in physical treatment and will therefore be restricted to a simple description of the functional problems. There are four factors to be considered in relation to physical treatment:

The type of involuntary movement.

The manner in which the involuntary movement disrupts the voluntary movement.

The degree of hypertonia.

The extent to which the emotional state influences movement.

(1) The type of involuntary movement is mentioned only to emphasize that it is almost irrelevant to physical treatment, which can not *directly* reduce involuntary movement.

(2) Involuntary movements can disrupt movement in two ways, acting separately or together: (*a*) the involuntary movement supersedes (superimposes itself on) the willed activity, which is distorted; (*b*) the involuntary movement disrupts the proximal fixation of a limb performing a willed movement. The movement cannot be performed adequately, without stable background posture.

(3) Although involuntary movements alone sometimes determine the disorder there is often associated hypo- or hypertonia, which implies disordered activity of tonic postural responses. Furthermore, proximal hypertonia (of the trunk and proximal limb joint muscles) may mask some of the involuntary movements for part of the time.

(4) Labile abnormal postures appear to be associated with a lack of emotional stability and disturbance of the emotions can release massive outbursts of involuntary movement activity. In some patients this phenomenon is so marked that their involuntary

TABLE 3

Primary Functional Difficulty: Type 2—Difficulty in Preventing (Involuntary) Movement (*see* p.37)

Involuntary movements distally	Involuntary movements proximally and distally	Involuntary movements with some spastic or plastic hypertonia	Spastic/plastic hypertonia with some involuntary movements	Variable posturing
Progressively greater effect of tonic responses ⟶				

movements appear to be caused almost solely by a failure to suppress the emotional influence.

Since physiotherapy can be directed only at certain elements of the disorder the classification is confined to these. Thus the various disorders can best be seen as being part of a spectrum (Table 3), with discreet involuntary movements at one end and, as the postural element gradually increases, gross postural changes at the other. It is appreciated that, whereas this classification may have no fundamental relevance for the physician, it has for the physiotherapist because it describes the various elements that we can or cannot treat. Some of those on the extreme right (Table 3) are in many ways more typical of the hypertonic group than the involuntary movement group so far as indications for treatment are concerned.

Difficulty in controlling a movement.   It is obvious that any child in the two earlier groups will have difficulty in controlling movements, but here we are concerned only with that small number whose difficulty in control is primary—the ataxias.

The term ataxia is popularly used to cover a wide range of disorders from ineptitude at games, untidy writing, clumsiness, and repeated falling, to inco-ordination so severe that the child can hardly perform any purposeful movement. It may also describe dysequilibrium, ataxic diplegia, ataxia with mild hypertonus, and ataxia with some involuntary movements. This wide variety of disorders can be subdivided into two groups:

(*a*) The type of movement mainly involved:
    (*i*) Gross postural movements.
    (*ii*) Fine movements.
    (*iii*) Both.
(*b*) Additional locomotor difficulties, if any:
    (*i*) Hypotonus.
    (*ii*) Hypertonus.
    (*iii*) Involuntary movements.

Classification by age of onset (*see* Table 1)

There are four pertinent groups:
(1) Congenital
(2) Acquired (*a*) in the first year; (*b*) between approximately one year and five years; (*c*) over five years.

A further subdivision of the last two acquired groups is helpful as it affects prognosis: (*i*) acquired less than one to two years previously; (*ii*) acquired two or more years previously

Congenital disorders.   These which, when non-progressive, constitute the majority of the cerebral palsies, are separated from the acquired lesions for two reasons: The baby has never had normal movements and therefore has not experienced the environment in a normal manner. He has no knowledge of the feel of certain movements or skills and perhaps only an imperfect, or distorted, understanding of the environment within which he is attempting to move. There is a possibility that parents' attitude to their baby will be different from one whose known normality was seen to be altered by illness or trauma. Since treatment of these children to a great extent involves the parents this is important.

Acquired disorders.   Most are of sudden onset, non-progressive and heralded by an acute episode during which the motor disorder is of little immediate concern. This is followed by a period of convalescence during which the motor sequelae appear only gradually, usually supplanting an initial flaccid stage. Next there is a period of approximately two years of gradual (but seldom complete) recovery.

Subdivision by age of onset is arbitrary but is reflected in the management.

Onset in the first year: in general these infants can be treated as though they have a congenital disorder once their motor defect has stabilized. They are most frequently hemiplegic. In theory the later the date of onset the better the chance of recovery, since they had a longer period of normal movement experience.

Onset between one year and five years: these have the advantage of previous sensory/motor experience and provided their lesion is not too severe they may re-learn many of their gross skills with comparative ease. They do not yet attend school and so it is likely that more time can be spared for physical re-education.

Onset over the age of five years: physiotherapy seems to have less to offer these than the younger children. Spontaneous recovery in a large number may foster extravagant claims for specific types of treatment. Despite such claims, the authors consider that, after the acute phase, specialized treatment techniques have yet to prove their worth in this field. This is not to say that the physiotherapist has no part to play. Her attitude of enlightened common sense towards rehabilitation is the greatest need during the two years following the onset of recovery.

(II) PHYSIOTHERAPY EXAMINATION

We shall refer only to the points peculiarly relevant to this type of movement disorder. It is based on the headings of Chapter 4 (1).

(a) Relevant facts not directly
    related to the movement
    examination
(b) Apparatus
(c) Orthopaedic surgery
(g) Other information

} None other than already mentioned in Chapter 4 (1)

(d) Deformity

In a disorder of movement and posture, postural deformity is not unnaturally a frequently presenting sign. Since any fixed deformity will follow the predisposing posture, some confusion of postural, fixed and structural deformity in this condition is inevitable.

Postural deformity. The postures, which are centrally determined but which need not be constant, are usually the result of contraction of the muscles noted below under 'fixed deformity'. When the posture is almost continuously maintained, fixed deformity frequently occurs and structural deformity may well follow.

Fixed deformity. Hypotonic and purely involuntary movement disorders are usually free from fixed deformity. Any hypertonia is likely to result in some muscle shortening. Typically the child who has hypertonia only will present with milder (but more symmetrical) contractures than one who has spasticity combined with athetosis. Common sites for significant muscle shortening are:

Upper limbs: Long finger flexors, thumb adductor and opponens, and forearm pronators.

Lower limbs: Hip: adductors, ilio-psoas
Hip/knee: rectus femoris, hamstrings
Knee/ankle: gastrocnemius
Ankle/foot: soleus, tibialis posterior, peronei

Structural deformity.   The hip joint is notoriously unstable in the congenital and the early acquired movement disorders. Both hypertonia and hypotonia can be the cause of subluxation and dislocation. Deformity of the femoral neck in hypotonic children presents as greatly increased external rotation of the hip in combination with limited internal rotation, probably as a result of the child's hip posture. True shortening of lower limb is relevant only in ambulant hemiplegia and asymmetric diplegia. It is suitably measured by placing graduated blocks under the shorter lower limb to level the pelvis.

Retention of the lumbar primary curve creates an effective kyphosis of the trunk and sometimes a compensatory lordosis of the cervical spine. Under-activity of the abdominal muscles or over-activity or contracture of the psoas major is the apparent cause of severe lumbar lordosis in some walking patients. Mild lateral curvature is comparatively frequent in asymmetrical disorders, but in our experience severe kypho-scoliosis is confined to the child with mixed spastic and athetoid cerebral palsy.

(e) Muscle power testing

Muscle power testing has little or no usefulness for two reasons. First, it is impossible to carry out the tests with any accuracy. Second, the power of the muscle has little relevance to the disorder of movement. As soon as a movement is 'cerebrally possible', the muscles concerned will strengthen themselves very quickly: this can be seen most dramatically after operation. Previously non-functioning dorsiflexor/evertor muscles can achieve full power within weeks of an elongation of the tendoachilles, because the operation has created a situation in which they can function. Unfortunately this sometimes happens after adductor tenotomy and obturator neurectomy, when the non-functioning abductors are suddenly activated leading to the opposite deformity. This latter group of children appear to have a strongly dystonic element in their movement disorder.

(f) Postural and movement ability

For clarity and simplicity our discussion of this will be restricted to gross movement abilities. If the disorder is mild the examination of those children, who are old enough and intelligent enough to follow instructions, can be straightforward. For younger, less intelligent or severely handicapped children there may be little 'voluntary' action in the examination.

Primitive and pathological responses (*see* Appendix 2). The physiotherapist will be interested in the presence or absence of responses such as hand and foot grasp, Moro, asymmetric tonic neck response, symmetric tonic neck response, tonic labyrinthine response and positive supporting reaction which will have become apparent during the previous examination. Also whether or not they are appropriate for the child's chronological and developmental age. To be significant these responses should be consistent enough to warrant the term 'reflex': indiscriminate response hunting is a sport which serves little purpose in physiotherapy.

Vertical suspension and the downward protective (parachute) response.   The response to this position and manoeuvre is important to the physiotherapist as it can be a guide to the future movement development the child will adopt. Approximately 10 per cent of infants have a tendency to prefer a 'supine' developmental sequence of sitting→shuffling→standing rather than the more usual 'prone' sequence of sitting→crawling→standing (13).

This minority of infants resists attempts to make them support their weight on extended legs until some months after they have learnt to shuffle and this trait (which appears to be dominantly inherited) is reflected in their persistent adoption of a 'sitting on air' posture in vertical suspension and to their having a modification or absence of the downward parachute response. The other protective responses need not be tested separately as they will have already been apparent during the gross movement examination.

Equilibrium reactions.   Reactions in sitting, all fours, kneeling and standing will have already been observed during study of the gross movements. Where relevant to treatment, prone and supine reactions will need to be tested separately.

Methods of recording the examination

Record keeping is an essential part of good treatment. It is however one thing to observe and assist a child's movement and to ask his parents about his abilities and problems at home and quite another matter to record this information in a useful manner. Many departments have devised their own charts and scoring methods. These certainly have a place, since they remind the staff to cover all the points, and can be a useful record. However, any chart tends to have one major drawback: the interesting and relevant details about a patient are so often those in which he differs from the others. It is because the differences are the most relevant items that most charts have large 'comments' columns and that the chart loses much of its purpose. For those (like the authors) who do not generally favour charts, the best method seems to be a concise description of abilities and disabilities in a set format.

(III) TREATMENT

The treatment of cerebral palsy and related movement disorders will be divided into three parts.

> Congenital and early acquired.
> Late acquired.
> Progressive conditions.

Each will be subdivided into headings:
Prevention of deformity.
Posture and movement.
Sensory stimulation.
Advice to parents.

In ideal circumstances an infant will be referred for treatment as soon as an abnormality is detected: for congenital disorders this is likely to be between six and twelve months and for the acquired disorders immediately following the acute episode.

It often happens that children are not referred for treatment until the early period of movement development is over and they may already have some fixed deformity. Each child presents different problems, but it should be appreciated that:

(1) Because children have not been having treatment in the past it may be possible to get some rapid improvement in function, but this does not imply that such great improvements will continue thereafter.

(2) There is a element of *fait accompli* about these children's disabilities and the neurodevelopmental treatment suitable for the

younger child may not for the older child be so effective, although it may (like any other approach) show some marked immediate benefits.

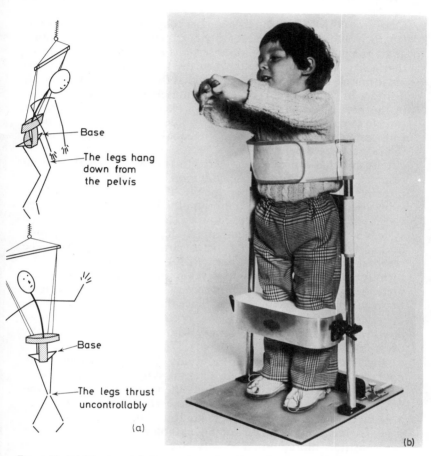

Figure 12. (a) The essential characteristic of standing is that the body weight is borne by the feet; it is not only that the body is vertical and the hips and knees straight. Bouncers or walking aids which suspend the infant by his pelvis, teach incorrect postural habits and so tend to increase rather than reduce the disability. Such walking frames do have a rôle in the management of some other disorders. (b) If a child is supported in standing, his plantigrade feet must form his base above which he supports his body. This can be achieved by manual support or by a standing frame. The frame shown has upright supports which are slightly flexible and so allow the child some postural adjustment of hips, knees and trunk whilst retaining a correct standing position

Congenital and early acquired disorders

Prevention of deformity

Sharrard (14) has pointed out that children's muscle/tendons lengthen as a consequence of bone growth, which by thrusting apart the muscles' origins and insertions applies a force to them; that a fixed deformity results when the forces applied to antagonistic muscle groups are unequal and that this occurs in a locomotor disorder in which there is differential muscle weakening. However, in the normal body, in spite of a marked disparity of available muscle strength across many joints, no deformities occur. It therefore seems unlikely that by itself unequal muscle strength can be the cause of fixed deformity.

It seems that muscle/tendon growth (or rather hypertrophy in response to bone growth) operates on a fundamental physical principle—le Chatelier-Braun principle, 'if any change of conditions is imposed on a system at equilibrium then the system will alter in such a way as to counteract the imposed change'. In this instance the system is the whole of the locomotor system required to maintain a normal posture at a joint and the constraint is bone growth. The cerebral palsy infant is not born with contractures or bony deformity but with a tendency to develop abnormal postures. These preferred postures imply *an abnormal ratio of muscle lengths* between opposing muscle groups. Since the same physical principle operates, muscle hypertrophy now occurs *so as to maintain the disorder of posture*. Thus a deformity, which was postural, gradually becomes fixed.

Any attempt to prevent fixed deformity by applying a 'constraint' upon the system is bound to fail, since the system will respond so as to retain its previous state. Therefore, the traditional splinting and passive stretching are self-defeating. Success can be achieved only by altering the system itself and there are three lines of approach:

(1) Exercises designed to inhibit pathological postural activity *and* substitute more normal activity. Such a treatment needs to be started early in the child's locomotor development (certainly by 6–9 months of age). It cannot be emphasized too strongly that the aim is not to strengthen muscles but to increase the likelihood of certain, previously unfavoured, movements occurring. In these disorders any muscle weakness is secondary to the disorder of posture.

(2) Splinting, which in this context is part of the child's movement

re-education and not, as often stated, designed to stretch a fixed deformity. The new posture produced by the splinting alters the proprioceptive input and so changes the output: this effectively alters the system. The method has limited applications, but is, nonetheless, of use. An example is in *postural* equinus: if the foot can be held at about 10 degrees of dorsiflexion, not only does the plantar flexor spasm cease but the dorsiflexors are activated. Thus a below-knee caliper with back stops on a well-fitted boot can be very effective when worn by a child just learning to stand and walk. We have never found night splints to be effective but consider that day splints do have an important role in the management of some children. Reluctance to prescribe splinting constitutes a contra-indication itself, as it is then used only as a last resort (which is too late) and by those who lack the experience to apply it to the correct patient, thereby confirming and reinforcing their reluctance. Splinting in cerebral palsy causes a strong division of opinion amongst physiotherapists, partly due to a sharp division in treatment methods: the mechanical versus the neurodevelopmental approach. The splint (whether a caliper, moulded support or plaster of paris) being the archetype of the mechanical approach is often abhorrent beyond reason to those favouring a neurodevelopmental treatment. Both sides have sound arguments, but these usually relate to differing circumstances and are in fact more complementary than antagonistic.

(3) Surgery is obviously the most direct method of altering the system. It is usually claimed that the purpose of surgery is to eliminate the fixed deformity and at the same time produce a balance of muscle strength across the joint, so as to maintain the correction. However, in cerebral palsy, the significant fact for maintaining correction is more likely to be the alteration of proprioception.

Bone and joint changes. The shape of bones and joints is determined in part by the use to which they are put, that is, the forces applied to them. Nowhere in the body is this more apparent than in the formation of the acetabulum and femoral head and neck. Gradual subluxation/dislocation of the hips is referred to elsewhere (*see* p.106) and when the cause is flexor and adductor hypertonus there is usually femoral neck ante-version and a failure of the femoral shaft/neck angle to decrease, frequently presenting as a marked increase in hip internal rotation at the expense of external rotation when tested with the hip in extension. There is sometimes little change in these ranges in flexion, and this difference is relevant to physical treatment. Children who sit between heel (*see Figure 51*), usually show the altered joint ranges of the hip in flexion and extension. However, it is standing rather than sitting which appears to be the key to combating this problem, i.e. correct and early weight bearing.

Whether the infant is (developmentally) ready to stand or not, weight bearing through extended hips should be started at about one year old. The feet should be plantigrade and the hips slightly abducted and rotated away from the position of deformity for that child. This exercise, together with measures later, may avoid severe hip joint deformity.

Bouncers (which stimulate the extensor thrust response of the lower limbs) are to be avoided at all cost, since they combine many disadvantages: not allowing full weight bearing, encouraging the deforming posture, and teaching that, as in sitting, his trunk is his base (from which his legs hang), whereas the very essence of standing is that the feet form the fixed point (*Figure 12*).

Limb shortening is significant only in the lower limbs, if it is asymmetric and for patients who are standing and walking. Its effects are varied. For a child with asymmetric diplegia, shortening may lead to some alteration of spinal posture, but more typically it has no spinal effect as it is compensated by an increased equinus of the shorter leg or an increased hip/knee flexion of the other. The hemiplegic patient may also compensate in this way, but more typically the pelvis drops on the affected side, causing a postural

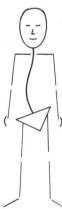

Figure 13. Lower limb true shortening may cause a compensatory lateral curvature of the spine

scoliosis concave to the opposite side (*Figure 13*). A lightweight heel (and perhaps sole) raise is needed if the shortening is greater than half an inch but it need not fully correct. Once fitted, a raise needs periodic checking for it may have no effect on posture, and growth may rapidly reduce or increase the true shortening.

Posture and movement

It is likely that more has been written about the treatment of posture and movement in cerebral palsy than on any other aspect of physiotherapy. A representative list of books and articles under 'Further Reading' will give the more interested reader good background information. There are many methods of treatment and the difficulties in describing the techniques have led to the use of eponyms. A discussion on treatment becomes a roll-call: Bobath, Brunnstrom, Collis, Doman, Kabat, Peto, Phelps, Rood, Temple Fay, Vojta. . . All the methods under these names 'work', some perhaps better than others all of the time and some better than others with certain patients and therapists. Lip service is given to eclectic treatment and, to a certain extent, all but the most rigid disciples of a method treat selectively. We consider that truly eclectic treatment (however desirable it may be) is not really possible for two reasons: (*a*) it takes a long time to become proficient at even one technique; and (*b*) the treatment must suit the physiotherapist as well as the patient: to be able to do all treatments equally well is probably to do them all equally badly.

It is difficult to appreciate a particular treatment method unless it has been practised for a time, for none should be judged from the rationale stated by its proponents. The majority of the methods grew out of empirical observations and the rationale was added later. As a general rule the more 'scientific' the explanation appears, the less the likelihood of its withstanding criticism: for these explanations often fail to take account of how crude our treatment methods are in relation to the physiological mechanisms expounded. Also, the more elaborate the treatment, the further it is removed from normality; and the ultimate aim of treatment is increased ability in ordinary life. It is not far from the truth to suggest that the explanations of treatment make sense only to those who already have a good working experience of the method.

It might seem reasonable to ask which system has the best results overall. It is difficult to judge for several reasons. The aims of treatments are sometimes different. Those who advocate one method might prefer it to be judged on prevention of fixed deformity, whilst to the proponents of an alternative method consideration of fixed deformity might be secondary to more normal patterns of movement. One method might be judged on the early age at which walking is achieved, while another might deliberately delay walking until it could be performed better. It is impossible to match children of equal handicap, for the handicap is not an isolated and direct result of the brain insult. It is a combination of this with all that has happened since. Hence, if two children, one treated and one untreated, have the same degree of handicap, it does not follow that treatment has not helped. Just as plausible an explanation is that the treated child would have been worse without treatment. Until means of more accurate early diagnosis (and therefore prognosis) and recording have been devised the influence of early treatment will remain unsettled. In the older age group, once the handicap has become established, the effects of different techniques can be judged more easily, but it does not follow that the treatments more successful at this age are also more effective in infancy. It would in fact seem unlikely, as the problems are different.

However, one approach to the treatment of these disorders is in a category by itself and not to single it out would be to present an unbalanced picture. The work of Dr and Mrs Bobath challenged the established treatments and influenced physiotherapy more than is often appreciated. Perhaps the highest compliment paid to them is that their teaching, once considered controversial, is now generally accepted and commonly incorporated in treatments bearing other names.

Treatment aims. Four causes of movement difficulty were described on page 35: hypertonus, hypotonus, involuntary movements, ataxia. A combination of causes may be found in one child. The means of treatment will vary with the child's movement difficulty, his age, intelligence and circumstances; but although the emphasis will change the underlying aims remain the same.

(1) To ensure that the child experiences a large choice of movement possibilities in a wide range of circumstances.

(2) To prevent the dominance of any postures or movements.

(3) To give experience of stable posture, from which movements can be performed.

(4) To give the child the opportunity to experience movement of his body as a whole to achieve an objective, i.e. to show him that co-ordinated movement is purposeful.

(5) To ensure that he appreciates responsibility for his body,

e.g. that his head is *his* and not something which is propped up by his mother's shoulder.

For the infant there may be little difference in emphasis of these aims, but as the child grows older it is likely that the following aims take priority:

Hypertonia (1) and (2)
Hypotonia (1), (3), (4) and (5)
Involuntary movements (3) and (4)
Ataxia (3) and (4)

The means of treatment are to create circumstances in which he can experience more natural movement (or posture). To begin with this may require that the movement be done for the child, to give him the sensation of it. This assistance will be withdrawn as quickly as possible so that he can carry out the movement on his own, though still in a position which makes it easier for him. Once he has achieved a movement the child is gradually given more and more difficult circumstances in which to achieve it, until (ideally) the movement can be performed in everyday situations. In point of fact this final stage will usually be accompanied by a falling off in the quality of the movement and part of the skill in treatment is to balance the quality of the movement with the difficulty of the situation in which it is performed.

Much of the treatment should employ the *balance and protective responses*. There are theoretical reasons for this, which are outside our scope here, but there are also sound practical reasons. Balance and protective responses utilize patterns of movement which are nearly always opposed to those preferred by the damaged brain, yet they can often be elicited without the voluntary assistance of the child. Consequently they are a particularly convenient method of widening the infant's and young child's movement experience (*see* Appendix 3).

As the child grows older the emphasis of treatment should gradually shift away from teaching new movements to the most economic and advantageous use of those he has. Much more of the available treatment time will be needed for training in daily living activities to allow greater independence. This is not because we consider that the previous treatment would not still give some benefit, but because the benefit of continuance of earlier treatments appears to be out of proportion to the time available and less worth while.

After any orthopaedic surgery an intensive treatment regime is well worth while as the operation should have altered the child's potential and opened up new avenues of movement.

Involuntary movements and ataxia. The early treatment of both these types of disorders is to ensure that the children get the maximum opportunity to experience normal movement and posture. This appears to be important and the authors consider it very desirable. However (*ignoring those with any hypertonic element*) intensive treatment of older children with involuntary movements and ataxia gives no benefit. Such children continue to improve gradually well into their 'teens by what may be a combination of late maturation, increased experience and greater determination and purpose. What they need is the opportunity to explore the limits of their ability in their everyday life. Learning new skills at a late age is not extraordinary in these children—it is natural, but it demands great persistence and courage from the child. It is for all those concerned with them to appreciate this and to sustain encouragement as well as providing the necessary opportunities.

Sensory stimulation

It has already been pointed out that cerebral palsy is a sensory as well as a motor disorder; proprioceptive experience being the key to motor ability. In this section the sensory stimulation referred to is mainly exteroceptive although, for an understanding of the environment, proprioception may sometimes be of equal or greater importance (e.g. appreciation of weight and object recognition).

From the earliest age the baby should be helped to feel his body: to play with his feet and legs, put his hands in his mouth, on his face and body and through his hair. If two-handed play is difficult, hand clasping and clapping as well as playing with toys and transferring them from hand to hand should be encouraged with only as much help as is needed. Toys should be of different colours, textures, sizes and weights as well as having a built-in noise (like a bell or a rattle). In this way an association between vision, hearing, touch and proprioception may be built up.

Experience of reaching out for a face or a toy to appreciate distance is needed. An understanding of distance is important, particularly the near-to (personal) space, not only to preclude secondary dysmetria but also for an appreciation of speed, which seems to require knowledge of a time: distance ratio. In this context it is interesting how often severely handicapped children with an over-active startle response shy away from a hand brushing hair out of their eyes or a spoon taking food to the mouth. Bearing in mind that they might have a better understanding of distance and speed from their own limbs, it is better to put the spoon in the child's hand and guide it to his mouth, even if he may never be likely to feed himself. In this way his proprioceptive experience can supplement his inadequate visual appreciation of the speed at which the object is approaching.

Experience of differing temperatures, textures, weights, colours, sounds and distances is important. Also percepts of above/below, inside/outside, behind/in front etc. can be introduced as part of dressing and bathing earlier than might be thought.

Parent advice

Those readers who are interested in detailed advice to help parents to understand and manage their children's movement disorders can refer to *Handling the Young Cerebral Palsied Child at Home* (15). Here the heading 'Parent Advice' is used to emphasize that, wherever possible, the treatment involves the training of parents in their child's everyday care. It is all day, everyday management, far more than hospital treatment by the physiotherapist, which will influence his sensory/motor development. However, the advice must be specific for the child and his particular circumstances. Some other aspects of parent advice have been dealt with in Chapter 2.

Late acquired disorders

Prevention of deformity

Most acquired disorders are of sudden onset and heralded by an acute episode during which the child may be unconscious or semi-conscious for some considerable time. Many such children make a comparatively good (movement) recovery, but during this period it is advisable to ensure that the child is not continuously in one preferred posture and to move joints through their full range daily. Once the child is able to sit up (in a bed or in a chair) all the usual considerations about chair sizes and posture will apply (*see* Appendix 6).

In those patients who are markedly spastic the tendency to fixed deformity can become severe and plaster of paris shells may be necessary. Where there is hypertonic quadriplegic involvement, deformity will seldom affect a child's locomotor abilities as recovery of voluntary function is not good, but this is no reason for ignoring the problem. At the very least a lack of fixed deformity will make nursing easier and the child more comfortable.

Prevention of fixed deformity in the hemiplegic child is important, regardless of the degree of spasticity. Good recovery is frequent and deformity (particularly in the lower limbs) can severely delay rehabilitation.

Posture and movement re-education

There seems little doubt that if movement ability is going to return it will do so on its own: if not, then nothing we can do will make it appear. Having seen many children do very well without help, we are opposed to *intensive* movement restoration regimes for most of these children. What usually happens is that an unconscious child gradually regains consciousness, being disorientated and with marked dysequilibrium, but improves over a two-year period to become a mildly ataxic, dysarthric (and usually cheeky) youngster. *Any* treatment carried out during that time would appear to have produced good results.

The physiotherapist should keep a watchful eye on the developing movement ability of the child and ensure that he has every opportunity to practise to their maximum those abilities which are returning. Without this supervision the authors have seen children left sitting in wheelchairs (usually adult size and hopelessly inadequate in every respect) for months after they could have been walking alone. It may take little more than an hour to 'teach' such a child to walk, because the necessary abilities are there already. The physiotherapist can prevent such failures to help. Her true role in this disorder is to ensure that those caring for the patient are aware of his gradual recovery, otherwise everyday highly protective attitudes to his social and motor abilities are likely to outlive the child's need of them. It is a different problem from the (apparently similar) adult situation.

Sensory experience

It has been suggested that sensory awareness should be encouraged even in the unconscious patient and there seems little reason to dispute this. It may well have some effect, takes little time and should be part of the routine physiotherapy of the unconscious patient. Deliberate efforts to stimulate vision, hearing and touch while the child remains semi-conscious and disorientated certainly have an effect, but whether the patient gains any long-term advantage has not been shown.

Advice to parents

Once the child is able to return home the parents may need help in daily living activities and advice about simple methods of promoting the child's abilities. Intensive exercises are seldom needed.

Progressive disorders

Physiotherapy has little to offer the child with a rapidly progressive degeneration of the higher centres of the central nervous system, though it helps parents to feel something practical is being done. Very slowly progressive disorders can be treated as cerebral palsy.

Prevention of deformity

The rapid progression of these conditions allows little time for structural deformity to develop but although prevention of fixed deformity serves no physical purpose, it may be of great comfort to the parents and give a feeling of doing something to help their child.

Posture and movement

In the central as opposed to the more peripheral degenerative disorders the children may rapidly develop severe mental limitation and if so attempts to maintain function are without purpose. It is better to give the parents (or the staff on the wards) advice on how the child can be made comfortable and nursed more easily.

Sensory stimulation

Serves no purpose.

Advice to parents

The parents may have been bringing the child up to a physiotherapy department regularly for treatment prior to the recognition that the condition was progressive. The physiotherapist may have come to know them very well and some parents like to continue coming (although less frequently). Treatment cannot forestall the outcome, but the comfort given by seeing the child and discussing his day-to-day problems is out of all proportion to the time required. This time should be found.

(b) THE SEVERELY SUBNORMAL CHILD

(I) PHYSIOTHERAPY EXAMINATION

This examination refers to points which are relevant only to un-complicated severe mental subnormality. It is based on the headings of Chapter 4 (1) and should read in conjunction with it.

(*a*) Relevant factors not directly related to the disorder
(*b*) Orthopaedic apparatus
(*c*) Relevant surgery
(*f*) Postural and movement ability
(*g*) Other information

No comments additional to Chapter 4 (1)

(*d*) Deformity

Structural deformity. Subluxation or dislocation of one or both hips is seen in children who adopt a frog posture (extreme flexion, abduction, external rotation of the hips with knee flexion). This is usually an anterior displacement of the femoral heads.

Fixed deformity. Any immobile child who is allowed to maintain the same posture over a period of years is at risk of developing alterations of muscle length and fixed deformity. It is interesting that it is not a constant finding. These 'contractures' are nearly always into flexion and common sites are elbows, fingers and thumb, knees and ankles (dorsiflexion).

Postural deformity. Usually a retention of infantile postures. Planovalgus feet are common in ambulant children and seem to be an exaggerated retention of normal infantile flat feet. They are due to hypotonia.

(*e*) Muscle power

Weakness (as opposed to hypotonicity) is not a problem of mental subnormality. There may be weakness secondary to inactivity, but it is never the factor preventing greater movement ability. Con-tinuous practice of stereotyped movements (or postures) may make them so easily elicited that they mimic spasticity. Typical of these movements is the supporting reaction producing total extension of the lower limbs when standing.

One purpose of the examination is to establish the movement

developmental age of the child so that a comparison may be made with his development in other fields. If his movement age is similar or older than his developmental age in other respects it is unlikely that physiotherapy will produce any increase in function. All the same it may be necessary to prevent habits of movement or contractures which might later prevent an increase of function. When movement ability lags behind other abilities the examination should be able to highlight the causative factors and suggest the steps needed to help him overcome them.

(II) TREATMENT AIMS FOR MOVEMENT DELAY IN THE SEVERELY SUBNORMAL CHILD

The problem of improving gross movement performance of severely retarded children *without a movement disorder* is complicated by their difficulty in breaking away from the movements they have already learned. These movement habits can be persistent to the extent of mimicking some aspects of hypertonic cerebral palsy. It is often considered that severely retarded children have poor protective responses and this has led some physiotherapists to concentrate on practising these deficient movements. We consider that the problem should be viewed the other way around: in addition to their ascribed function the protective responses can be seen as postural mechanisms of changing position or exploration (*see* Appendix 3). This is how they are normally used by an infant in getting from lying to sitting, sitting to crawling, crawling, cruising and walking. If the child lacks the desire to move about, he does not use this type of movement but instead practises the 'static' equivalent of balancing on a fixed base. The problem then is one of increasing the *desire* to move, not the ability: for a lack of ability would imply a *disorder* of movement.

Our aims must therefore be:

(1) To ensure that the child experiences a wide range of postural and movement opportunities and so prevent the dominance of one pattern.

(2) To encourage exploratory movements. Since such a child has previously shown little desire to move towards a rewarding situation (either because he cannot appreciate the reward or has learnt that it will eventually come to him) it seems appropriate to reverse the situation by making his present position uncomfortable, or at least unrewarding. Unstable or 'half-way' positions are ideal for this: for

instance a child who will happily lie prone or supine all day may move out of a side lying position: a child who will sit contentedly on the floor, may move into a crawl position, or get to kneeling or standing if taken half-way towards the position. These positions are designed to be uncomfortable only so long as he makes no effort to move out of them, and to be rewarding once he has.

Perhaps it needs saying and should be emphasized that the treatment should not be painful. There is no need to hurt. It may be argued that these children would respond to bribes quite as well—and that this would be better—but our experience of young severely mentally handicapped children cannot support such a view.

(3) To make him appreciate his 'responsibility' for his body. This aim is closely related to aim (2), but we think needs emphasizing from this different standpoint. All too often children are placed in totally supported positions (whether lying or sitting) and one gets the impression that the most stimulating time of their life was *in utero*. Total support may be all that can be achieved for some children, but many can benefit from periods in a less comfortable environment. For example a chair which supports them only where necessary (*see* Appendix 6) or a prone-lying ramp to stimulate head extension and arm support.

(4) To give him an opportunity to experience a wide range of 'toys'—not the usual mass of plastic objects which mean something only to an adult. Instead of these, a child should have a selection of real household objects of different size, colour, weight and texture with perhaps a set of one inch cube 'bricks' to pick up.

(5) To train him to be independent as possible—even if it is no more than lifting an arm or a leg to co-operate in dressing.

(6) To stimulate communication, which inevitably occurs during a treatment session.

(c) SPINA BIFIDA CYSTICA

Introduction

Energetic primary treatment of spina bifida presents a new challenge to many physiotherapy departments. Since the physical treatment is closely allied with the orthopaedic management, and must be tailored to complement it, there are several approaches to physical treatment.

No one has many years' experience of treating large numbers of spina bifida children. Only now are there affected adolescents in any number and it is likely that they represent a different population from those who survived previously. In spite of devoted care and vigorous treatment, many are wheelchair-bound and have rejected the calipers and appliances which they tolerated when younger. It is salutary to consider that the children usually want to walk, but the available apparatus has such limited potential that their best achievement can in no way be compared to real walking. They can keep up with their peers more easily when in a wheelchair. As occurs sometimes in paediatrics, the patients have had to grow up before the inadequacy of the treatment was appreciated. Now that the need has been realized, bio-engineers in a number of centres are trying to improve caliper efficiency, but it may be several years before any improvements are generally available. From the beginning all surviving infants are given every encouragement towards independence.

The physiotherapy is not complicated in itself, but it becomes so because of the number of problems presented by each child. The clash of priorities can be inconvenient. 'Team-work' (a popular phrase in chronic neurological disorders) is essential in spina bifida and each member has to modify his ideal treatment so as to dovetail in with reality. Therefore physical treatment is rarely as straightforward as it might appear from the outline which follows, and for this reason a brief comment on some of these other factors is necessary.

(I) FACTORS LIKELY TO DELAY OR MODIFY PHYSIOTHERAPY

Congenital spinal/thoracic structural deformity

Hemivertebrae, absent or deformed ribs, scoliosis and kyphosis all influence the physiotherapist's task. Treatment time will be lost by extensive surgery; the child may be prevented from developing efficient use of his arms; and thoracic supports for calipers will have to be modified. The child's general health may be the worse because of reduced respiratory function and the distortion of his mediastinal organs.

Lower limb deformities

The most important factor to remember is that the deformities are not static and will alter with growth. Constant reassessment and replanning of therapy is necessary, as what appeared trivial at 12 months may have become a much more significant handicap at three years.

Dislocated hips will not necessarily modify the therapist's task (the distribution of muscle power is more important) for it may be quite practical to fit calipers and establish an acceptable walking pattern when *both* hips are displaced. Fixed flexion of the hips and fixed flexion or recurvatum of the knees can rarely be resolved by physiotherapy alone. A variety of foot deformities may be encountered, which complicates shoe fitting, and therefore progress towards walking in calipers.

Sensory loss

Some sensory loss is inevitable, therefore calipers need to be carefully fitted and padded. Great care is necessary when strapping is used for correction of deformities. Shoes and clothes must fit well, to minimize the likelihood of pressure sores.

Fractures

Pathological fractures occur in spite of vigilant care, most often following long immobilization in plaster, and every effort should be made to reduce immobilization time. Fractures should never prevent activity, as they are usually simple fractures without displacement, easily protected by pressure bandages, back-slabs or plaster cylinders. Physiotherapy is not interrupted.

The authors have no conclusive evidence that exercise will reduce the incidence of fracture although it is a reasonable supposition which has general support (16).

Incontinence

Surgery. Ileal loop operations are often desirable and necessary, but surgery and recovery interrupt the rhythm of physical treatment and subsequently time is spent regaining lost ground. Surgical operations complicate the fitting of suitable trunk and lower limb braces so that pre-operative consultation to ensure optimal siting of the stoma is essential.

Hydrocephalus

Surgery for insertion or replacements of a valve interrupts physiotherapy and the presence of a valve alters some aspects of treatment.
In addition, children with hydrocephalus may present with:

(1) Cerebral palsy   } which will complicate treatment
(2) Mental subnormality } and limit the child's abilities

(II) PHYSIOTHERAPY EXAMINATION

Examination of the infant with spina bifida concentrates mainly
on his disabilities. As the child grows, particularly from one year
onwards, the emphasis shifts to his developing abilities. Thus, the
early records of a child will be concerned with:

Lack of function, both motor and sensory
Structural, fixed and postural deformity
Hydrocephalus and its sequelae

Whereas, later on, will be added:
General movement ability
Any specific features delaying progress

Assessing the disability

In many hospitals the physical assessment is carried out by the
physiotherapist, and opinion varies on how extensive it need be.
The immediate concern is to establish the approximate level of the
lesion, which is the main guide to the infant's prognosis since it
dictates:

(1) The extent of the paralysis.
(2) The distribution of sensory loss.
(3) The type of fixed deformities likely to appear.

Paralysis

Neonates and infants up to one year: assessment from the earliest
age has been shown to be reliable in most instances. Neonatal
reflexes and responses can be used and muscles which are functioning
noted. At this stage it is not always possible to grade individual

muscle power accurately and perhaps 'strong', 'weak' or 'absent' is best. It may be unwise to translate these into M.R.C. (*see* p.70) scale numbers as it implies a standard of precision which is usually impossible to achieve.

Child: more accurate muscle strength testing is possible, but this is seldom as simple as it may seem. Charts of children under three years should be interpreted with caution even when compiled by an experienced examiner. Wherever possible charting should be repeated by the same therapist on a separate occasion. Testing muscles individually may be essential for pre-operative assessment but seems to serve little purpose for a general assessment where the power of muscle *groups* may give all the information needed. These should be graded on the M.R.C. scale.

Sensory loss

Neonates and infants: The level of sensory loss helps to confirm the motor assessment by demonstrating the upper level of the lesion. It is important to note not only whether there is any reaction to a sensory stimulus but also whether the baby has appreciated it at cortical level for the response may represent a spinal reflex only.

Child: it is essential to note sensory loss so that precautions may be taken when using apparatus.

Fixed and postural deformity

These are typical of the level of the lesion, since they are usually caused by muscle imbalance. Accurate angular measurement of joint ranges is always difficult—particularly in babies, for whom 'severe', 'mild' and 'none' is the best classification.

Spine: with thoracic or thoraco-lumbar lesions there is always the likelihood of fixed deformity developing when the child sits or stands (in calipers). Congenital structural abnormalities have already been mentioned. High kyphosis is usually associated with a poor prognosis so far as physical achievement is concerned and this must be considered carefully when making long-term plans.

Hips: dislocation is frequent with paralysis below L.3 or 4 and likely to develop if below L.1 or 2. Fixed deformity of flexion, combined with adduction or abduction, often occurs.

Knees: hyperextension is frequently seen with lesions below L.3

or 4. Fixed flexion deformities are found in some neonates with lesions above L.1 or 2.

Ankles and feet: equino varus, calcaneo varus/valgus are all seen.

Assessing abilities

The infant and young child: includes an assessment of the upper trunk strength and balance (particularly in sitting), general activity and interest in movement. This is essential information when deciding upon the appropriate time to start caliper training.

The older child: postural and movement ability in three situations: (*i*) without bracing; (*ii*) with bracing; and (*iii*) self-help—particularly bracing.

(i) and (ii) A general assessment of ability as described in (*f*) on page 34.

Upper limb function is extremely important, particularly the strength of those movements needed for using crutches and propelling a wheelchair. The children's ability to get on and off a prone trolley, a Chailey Chariot, or a wheelchair is noted. When assessing the gait of a child using full-length calipers (particularly with a pelvic or thoracic band) it is not enough to watch him walk on a smooth level floor. He should be seen going up and down slopes and steps, walking outside on uneven ground, and his endurance must be noted. This may, in the end, be the factor determining whether or not calipers are of real use. Slow walking is time-consuming and can be the cause of endless frustration to the family, particularly the more conscientious, who feel that walking practice is essential.

(iii) Apart from the usual self-help activities such as dressing, a record should be made of the child's ability to put on and take off his calipers, and his interest and co-operation in looking after them.

(III) TREATMENT

The physical treatment of children with myelomeningocele can be divided into:

    Early (baby) treatment
    Later treatment

Each is subdivided into four sections:

    Correction/prevention of deformity
    Posture and movement
    Sensory
    Advice to parents

Early (baby) treatment

Correction/prevention of deformity

This is the most important early activity of the physiotherapist. There is little doubt that if this part of the treatment is delayed, or not given full priority, much additional orthopaedic surgery will be required. This is not only unfortunate for the child, but also absorbs time which could be put to better use. Much has been made of the danger of fractures *caused by manual stretching* to correct these deformities but, provided the physiotherapist is aware of this consequence of over-enthusiasm, the danger is more a myth than a menace.

It is a good rule to move all joints through their full range every day. There is then no danger that insidious fixed deformity will be overlooked. This is followed by stretching those joints which have a fixed deformity. Some deformities are too rigid for manual correction and for these either splinting or traction will be required. The skin in these areas is almost certain to be anaesthetic and therefore great care is taken to instruct the parents in general skin care. However, anaesthetic skin is not a contraindication to correctly applied strapping. We favour the Robert Jones strapping (*see Figure 16*) for talipes equino varus and have not been troubled by skin breaking down or fractures. Considerable skill is needed and parents should not be asked to do their child's strapping.

The head shape of the infant is readily affected by its habitual posture, particularly when there is an hydrocephalus. Head shape is important cosmetically and also functionally, for the 'normal' head is well balanced in relation to the disposition of its controlling muscles. Severe deformity can increase the difficulty of learning head control, particularly in a child who has inadequate trunk and lower limb fixation.

Most infants with a Spitz–Holter valve prefer to lie with the side of the head containing the valve uppermost. This preferred posture will produce an elongation of antero-posterior head length and a decrease in width. It may also produce skewhead (plagiocephaly). Until the infant's back has healed it may be impossible to avoid side lying, but, once healed, he should be generally nursed supine and some means of support, either sand bags or a head rest should be used. Deformity can be avoided by the use of foam templates, which are simple, cheap to make and disposable. They require careful supervision in case the baby vomits.

Some spinal deformities can be lessened by physiotherapy.

(1) By encouraging back extension, giving the child plenty of prone activity.

(2) By ensuring that the child's back is well supported either by muscle power or external aid, and that he is never just propped up in a pram or cot on soft pillows, or placed in a chair which has too upright a backrest.

However, the problem is often so great that the benefit is minimal.

Posture and movement

The body moves as a unit. Paralyse any part of it and *all* movements are affected to some extent: paralyse a large part and this has a significant effect. A prime mover requires a stable origin, but each muscle origin must itself be stabilized by its own fixators or synergists: this chain of stability is lost at the paralysed segment. Thus even the most early developmental movements are affected. These infants need help when learning to move and very definitely benefit from it.

For the first few days the neonate requires no *movement* physiotherapy: he is in no condition for being moved around, nor is there any need. As soon as possible (usually when the back has healed) head control and forearm support lying prone should be encouraged. He can be helped in this by firm pressure on his buttocks to stabilize his back and neck extensors or by support of his thorax and shoulder girdle (*Figure 14a, b, c*). Rolling may need help as it is hindered if his legs cannot contribute. Maintaining and achieving sitting is difficult without pelvic stability and any supports provided will need to take account of his head control and spinal deformity.

Sensory

There are two problems which concern us as follows:

(1) Sensory loss has to be borne in mind throughout treatment: strapping, plaster of paris, clothes and moving around on the floor can be dangerous.

(2) Sensory experience is not so likely to be limited in these as some other congenitally handicapped children. Nevertheless, it is advisable to ensure that toys are near the infant and that he is encouraged to reach for them. His general immobility will immediately deprive him of some sensory experience and this can be counteracted by imaginative play.

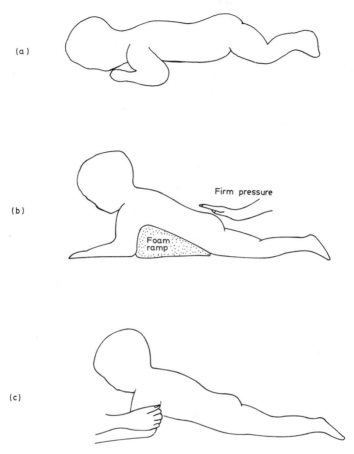

Figure 14. Assisting a child with spina bifida to be more effective when lying prone. (a) A lack of adequate (muscle) fixation will cause movement disability in parts of the body where there is no disorder. (b) Manual fixation of the pelvis allows effective use of the spinal extensors. A ramp under the chest makes it easier. (c) Manual fixation of the shoulder girdle and upper arms allows experience of head control

Advice to parents. When he is discharged home for the first time it will probably be the responsibility of the ward sister to advise the parents on all normal day-to-day care of the baby. The physiotherapist needs to explain the physical treatment to be carried out at home, such as daily stretching and manipulation. She will explain why these are necessary and check that the parents can carry them out. Some exercises will also be shown and the parents should be given a list of all that they have to do at home. They are *the* most important members of the treatment team, but need to be carefully instructed to achieve their maximum efficiency.

Later treatment

Correction and prevention of deformity

After the neonatal and early infant period, physiotherapy cannot assist in the correction of fixed deformity. This is in the hands of the orthopaedic surgeon. Immediate pre-operative physiotherapy is entirely concerned with an assessment of the child's abilities and their limitation due to deformity. Post-operative physiotherapy is directed towards:

(1) Maintaining improved joint range.
(2) Mobilizing stiff joints following immobilization.
(3) Re-educating muscle transplants.
(4) Training gait pattern. This may have altered and so need different apparatus from that of the pre-operative stage. In some instances the aim of surgery is to decrease the amount of bracing necessary.

By their very nature spontaneous fractures cannot be prevented. Simple splinting alone is usually adequate treatment and should not interrupt activity.

Posture and movement

It is desirable to begin standing by about 12 months: but this age is very much modified by the child's 'inclination'. The aims of standing are to:

(1) Enable the child to appreciate his surroundings from a more normal position.
(2) Give the lower limb bones and joints an opportunity to adapt to weight bearing.
(3) Improve lower limb circulation.
(4) Improve renal, bladder and bowel function.

Early standing may be encouraged with manual support, simple back-slabs or a standing frame. Any child with a lesion above L.4 will require some form of bracing very early on. Full-length calipers will maintain knee extension, but to stabilize the hips and trunk a pelvic band and thoracic support will be needed. (For further information on calipers, *see* Appendix 5.)

Standing and walking practice progress together, from firm supports such as parallel bars to walking aids, quadrapods and elbow crutches.

Strong arms are important for manoeuvring a wheelchair, transferring from a chair to a bed etc., and usually for support when standing. Therefore, every child has a regimen of exercises for his trunk, shoulder girdle and arm muscles (*Figures 15a and b*) initiated from the very beginning of a treatment programme.

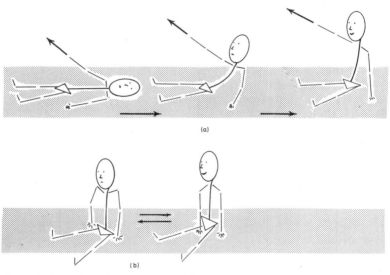

Figure 15. *The independence of a spina bifida child may depend on strong arms. Shoulder girdle and arm exercises are an essential part of the early physical management. (a) Pulling to sitting with one hand only, to encourage the infant to push up with the opposite arm. (b) The child lifts himself by elbow extension and shoulder girdle depression: strengthening the muscles needed later for support when walking*

As the children get older, greater emphasis should be placed on preparing them for an independent adult life. For many, full independence will be impossible, but each child will be helped to achieve his own maximum potential. This is likely to be limited more by his intellect and personality than his physical disability, provided he has had early and continued physiotherapy supervision and encouragement.

Sensory

Skin care. As the children approach adolescence and adulthood, they must be encouraged to take over the supervision of skin care themselves. With increased weight, trophic ulcers become a greater danger. A skin breakdown may develop as a result of a few moments' negligence—for example, a wrinkled sock in a tightish shoe—but may take months to heal, thereby restricting activity and causing great frustration. Vulnerable areas—heels, toes and sites where calipers touch the skin—must be inspected regularly.

Suitably sited mirrors low down on a wall are a simple aid to self-help. If an ulcer does occur pressure must be removed and vigorous treatment started immediately. Large doses of ultra-violet radiation (*see* Appendix 7) will help, as will ice-packs, other means of cold therapy and various special dressings. Ice has the advantage of being a possible means of home treatment. The authors suspect however, that it is constant attention which is the most important factor in any of these treatments.

Proprioception. Proprioception is essential for normal motor control. When the muscles related to a joint are paralysed the patient is deprived of the muscle feedback and, in most instances, that from the ligaments as well.

Advice to parents

Advice must be constantly available and geared to each family's individual needs. Initially frequent discussions and training sessions will be necessary as the amount of information which can be absorbed and retained during the first stressful months is limited. Later on, the family may learn to accept their child and need little advice except at times of surgery or appliance fitting. The important thing is that when a problem arises the parents know where they can obtain understanding and constructive advice.

Currently, much thought is being given to the future treatment of spina bifida following the experience of the last decade. It is our belief that whatever decisions are reached, every surviving baby should have the opportunity of immediate and continued intensive physiotherapy.

(d) PERIPHERAL NEUROMUSCULAR DISORDERS

(I) THE PHYSIOTHERAPIST'S EXAMINATION

(*a*) Relevant facts not directly related to
    movement examination
(*b*) Apparatus
(*c*) Surgery
(*d*) Deformity
(*f*) Postural and movement ability
(*g*) Other information

No comments
additional to
Chapter 4 (1)

(*e*) *Muscle power*

Muscle power is likely to be the most important aspect determined by the examination. Not only is the information of interest in itself, but in peripheral disorders (unlike some movement disorders of higher origin) it has a direct relationship to the child's function. Depending on the cause of the disorder and the purpose of the examination there are basically two ways of testing muscle power:

(1) By the strength of a movement, e.g. flexion of the forearm at the elbow.

(2) By the strength of individual muscles, e.g. (for elbow flexion) biceps brachii, brachialis, brachio-radialis, common flexor origin muscles.

In Great Britain the standard method of measurement is the *Medical Research Council Scale* (10):

0 = No contraction
1 = Flicker or trace of contraction
2 = Active movement with gravity eliminated
3 = Active movement against gravity
4 = Active movement against gravity and resistance
5 = Normal power

It is more difficult to assess muscle power in children than adults, but progression from 4 to 5 may be as inevitable as going out to play. In a deteriorating condition it is perhaps best to err on the optimistic side. Doing this is likely to show up the distribution of any muscle weakness more clearly, as some of the reduced strengths may be secondary to enforced inactivity.

Although it is very tempting to elaborate the system with plus and minus, the authors consider that such an elaboration of the scale takes away all its attraction. It is better to have the same person (with her own set of standards) testing the child each time and keeping to the 0–5 scale. However there is one exception to this rule which seems necessary: the gap between 3 and 4 is so great, and covers such an important range of ability, that 3+ seems essential.

(II) PERIPHERAL NEUROMUSCULAR DISORDERS: CLASSIFICATION AND TREATMENT AIMS

The disorders may be temporary or permanent, acute, chronic or progressive. From the point of view of physical treatment they can best be divided into two groups:

(A) Those which will not get worse and may get better

(B) Those which are inevitably progressive

Within Group (A) are of course many types of conditions affecting the various neuromuscular components. The differences will alter the emphasis of the aims and means of treatment. In this chapter we are giving an overall view: in Section II particularly relevant points will be listed under each condition together with references to the detailed treatment.

The significance of classifying peripheral neuromuscular disorders into two groups only can be summed up by the following questions:

First, are we maintaining the locomotor system in good order so that it can be effective when recovery takes place, as in A; or to maintain the best possible function, as in B?

Second, are we attempting to improve any muscle activity there is, as in A; or maintain it for as long as possible, as in B?

Third, should we be placing restrictions on the child's present life so that he will lead a fuller life when older, as in A; or should we rather be considering his enjoyment of the present, as in B?

Treatment will be considered under three headings:

(1) Deformity.

(2) Movement.

(3) Sensory loss.

GROUP A CONDITIONS

Deformity

Causes (*i*) intrinsic soft tissue contracture, for example, myositis; (*ii*) muscle imbalance and/or gravity; (*iii*) unequal bone growth; (*iv*) immobility

Intrinsic soft tissue contracture may occur while there is an active disease process affecting the motor unit. The measures are therefore short-lived and also as much a part of nursing as physiotherapy. The aim of treatment at this stage is to allow full-range passive movements of the affected joints, and this will entail measures to reduce pain and protective spasm. This can be achieved by supporting the limb, and heat (which has the additional advantage of increasing the circulation to the area).

In spite of these measures full-range passive movements may not be possible because of pain and muscle spasm.

Muscle imbalance and/or gravity. The impression is sometimes given that the musculo-skeletal system is a wilful producer of deformity: that if given any chance it will produce a distortion. This is far from true: its peculiar facility is to adapt itself to the use that is made of it, particularly while it is still growing. Once a disease process is finished, deformity may be caused by muscle imbalance but only when there is a maintained deviation in normal posture. This can be caused in three ways by:

(1) Muscle spasm: (*see* pp. 46–47).

(2) Gravity: support must be provided whenever posture is habitually altered by the unopposed pull of gravity. Typical sites are the vertebral column (by far the most important, as full surgical correction of the deformity is unlikely), and all joints in the lower limb. This will involve the use of spinal supports and calipers. Posture in bed can be the cause of fixed deformity. Night splints or support may be needed, particularly at the ankle, one of the few sites where gravity can have a detrimental effect in bed.

(3) Muscle action: muscles do not act solely to produce movement (concentric action) and to maintain posture. Equally important is their eccentric action: checking movements, absorbing excess kinetic energy. For example, when walking the hamstrings prevent the inertia of the lower leg from hyperextending the knee at the end of the swing phase. If the hamstrings are ineffective, genu recurvatum may result.

Unequal bone growth is seen usually when there has been a

massive denervation of one limb only. It is significant in the lower limb as it makes walking unsightly and inefficient and may tilt the pelvis to one side leading to a compensatory scoliosis (*see Figure 13*).

Immobility. The purpose of a joint is to allow movement: deprived of this function it will, in the presence of other pathological changes, become less efficient. Whenever possible total immobility should be avoided by taking the joint through its full range of movement at least once a day.

Movement

In all Group A conditions this refers to methods of re-educating muscles to work with greater:
(1) Strength.
(2) Endurance.
(3) Co-ordination.
Of these co-ordination is by far the hardest and the one least appreciated by those not directly involved. A physiotherapist will have little difficulty helping a child achieve strength and endurance, but her skill, patience and tenacity will be stretched to their limit achieving co-ordination—or rather in managing to coax from the child all his tenacity, patience and courage. Fortunately this aspect of treatment becomes important only when there is massive loss of function. Today this is rare in any country with good medical (and therefore physiotherapy) services.

When there has been a peripheral nerve injury several months may elapse before the muscle can function again. Meanwhile the tissue should be maintained in good condition. Electrical stimulation of the muscle tissue itself by long-duration pulses is not feasible with children as it is uncomfortable and not well tolerated. Increasing the circulation to that area could help but, in practice, children's muscle tissue seems more viable than adult's and does not appear to need these measures. It *is* important to prevent overstretching and some means of splinting may be required.

Strength. There is a variety of methods in use for re-educating muscle strength—perhaps the most popular at the moment being proprioceptive neuromuscular facilitation. In the authors' experience this method is not very successful with young children as, unless modified, it needs a large degree of patient co-operation. All methods of exercise, however, are attempts to get the maximum excitation at the anterior horn cells. This requires a high level of stimulation such as encouragement, traction or compression of joints, the muscle stretch reflex and recruitment by activating muscles which are already strong. To begin with all the movement may have to be done by the physiotherapist with the muscle just flickering in co-operation. Gradually this help will be reduced and subsequently replaced by resistance (gravity, manual, weights or springs).

Endurance. Strength is said to be increased by working intermittently against a near maximum load: endurance by working more continuously against a much smaller load. Children are usually not so inhibited as adults and use whatever muscle power is available to them. Exercises to increase endurance are not necessary.

Co-ordination. In the normal course of events the co-ordination of muscle action is not disturbed to an extent which could benefit from physical treatment. With peripheral nerve injuries certain muscles will recover function earlier than others and movement returning to a segment of a limb will be inco-ordinate for a time, but this is of little significance.

However in poliomyelitis when the interneurone pool may have been damaged the problem is real for co-ordination is disturbed at spinal level and the physiotherapist must re-educate movement away from the automatic, but inco-ordinate, patterns.

Sensory loss

Peripheral nerve lesions are usually accompanied by some loss of sensation. Although it is seldom a problem, greater care needs to be taken of the skin in the affected area and any supportive splinting should be more frequently checked. Where the nerve injury is combined with a fracture particular vigilance will be needed to prevent pressure sores from the plaster of paris—but in the normal course of events this *should* not be the physiotherapist's responsibility.

GROUP B CONDITIONS (*See* page 71)

Deformity

Many of the children present a massive challenge which is hard to meet. Fixed deformities of the hips and knees and equinus feet almost inevitably develop once the child is off his feet and into a chair-bound life. Daily passive stretching may decrease or delay their development and should be carried out because the deformities make nursing very difficult. The prognosis for the progressive conditions makes it hard to justify putting the child to too much discomfort and inconvenience with more elaborate means of prevention, which are bound to limit the mobility he retains.

Deformity of the upper limb is unlikely to be a factor limiting the child's ability and causes only slight nursing difficulty.

As usual, the trunk is a major problem and the physiotherapist has little to offer (but *see* p. 116). If the child is to lead any sort of active life he will have to sit and gravity will inevitably take its toll. Some form of spinal support to prevent a kyphoscoliosis may be used and should be checked periodically for condition and fit. So should the chair in which he sits.

Movement

It is generally agreed that specific measures to strengthen muscles in these conditions serve no purpose, provided the child has been given the opportunity to use his body to the best of his abilities. It is considered harmful to fatigue muscles and the child should be left to find *his own level of activity within a stimulating environment,* which must somehow be provided. Because gravity is often the big enemy, swimming (perhaps in the guise of hydrotherapy) can be both enjoyable and effective. The role of the physiotherapist is to ensure that:

(1) The child has a chair which supports him correctly both at home and at his day nursery or school. This is essential if he is to maintain the maximum opportunity to play and learn.

(2) He has suitable means of locomotion: i.e. suitable for his age, ability, environment and opportunity to use his available muscle power. As a young child, crawling/creeping, walking with or without support, or the use of a Chailey Chariot (*see* p. 130), tricycle or pedal car may be best; giving him the opportunity to transfer from one method to another as play and circumstance demand and to utilize varying muscle groups to their best advantage. As he grows he will need a wheelchair and there may well come a time when his muscle power is altogether insufficient for him to get about and a powered chair will be needed.

Sensory loss

Sensory loss is not usually a feature of these conditions.

3. ORTHOPAEDIC SITUATIONS

(a) PRE- AND POST-OPERATIVE ASSESSMENT

Where a close relationship exists between the orthopaedic and physiotherapy departments, much of what might be considered to be orthopaedic assessment is carried out by a physiotherapist. The fact that this co-operation has worked so well in many hospitals should encourage others. Many children are not seen at their best (or truest) in the usual rush of an outpatient clinic, whereas in the physiotherapy department there may be time for the child to relax and co-operate in a full assessment. The information needed by the surgeon will vary from child to child but can be discussed under the following headings:

Speculative

The opportunity for a full examination of a child's movement ability allows tentative answers to questions such as: what could be limiting his movement ability? Could it be generalized muscle weakness, muscle imbalance, dysequilibrium, inco-ordination, or the presence of fixed deformity? If these deficiencies were absent or reduced, would his performance be better? Are there contributing (and perhaps more important) factors such as mental retardation or visual defects? The fact that a physiotherapist is not qualified to test the level of intellect or visual acuity is of little importance here: she *is* uniquely qualified to assess movement ability and, implicitly, recognize the difference between a movement disorder due to a direct locomotor cause and movement disorder due to other causes.

With the knowledge of the bracing and surgical procedures available, and experience of their effects on past patients, it is possible to consider the effects they might have on the child being assessed. For instance, if a child's legs could be straightened (by bracing or surgery) would it help him to stand and walk? For this it is necessary to know whether he can balance and use his arms for support; whether he has reached the (movement) developmental age to stand, and is likely to want to. This information can be summarized in a report for the surgeon and should help him to make his decision. Ideally there should be discussion with the physiotherapist Both will profit from this.

Information relevant to surgery

When the aim of surgery is to alter the action of a muscle—usually by moving one of its attachments—it is often useful for the surgeon to know not only its power but also that of the other muscles acting over the same joint(s). The authors' view on the relevance of muscle power testing in cerebral palsy or similar disorders is discussed on p. 42.

A record of function

It is useful, and interesting, to be able to compare the level of pre- and post-operative function. Testing has two parts:

Functional ability tests. These are the more important tests when surgery is to improve the child's physical ability, rather than appearance. Tests will naturally vary with the type and site of surgery, but should be relevant to everyday activities.

Isolated tests. These usually include recording joint ranges, muscle shortening and power, and limb shortening. Spinal deformity is better measured from x-rays and this is not the physiotherapist's concern.

(b) PRE- AND POST-OPERATIVE TREATMENT*

For some years, both authors carried out pre- and (more particularly) post-operative general exercises on patients in their care. We had been taught that the child would benefit. This belief is yet another instance of adult treatment attitudes being transferred to children. There is little doubt that adults benefit from a regime of general exercises when in bed or chair-bound. It is not unreasonable to consider that the older the patient the greater the benefit. Children

---

* Pre-and post-operative respiratory treatment is discussed on pp. 27–28

usually move any part of their body which is not firmly fixed, and often parts we imagine to be. In fact, while in bed, they exercise themselves.

Out of bed, or out of plaster, things are different. Whilst there seems little place for intensive treatment in the physiotherapy department, there is often a need for a careful analysis of the child's difficulty as he explores his way towards the increased function which the operation has offered him. From such an analysis a simple statement of specific treatment aims can be made and a few exercises or games devised. There is often good reason for the treatment to be carried out in the physiotherapy department but, more frequently, the exercises are shown to the parents who can then do them with the child at home. The parents may be asked to bring the child up to the hospital at regular intervals for a check on his progress, alteration of the exercises and modification of any apparatus he is using. It is important that the aims of each exercise should be explained to the parents.

Anxieties about the results of surgery

In spite of pre-operative discussions, many parents are very worried because their child has not shown an immediate improvement after surgery and a brief repetition of the pre-operative explanation that the full benefits of that particular operation may take several months to be seen is reassuring. It must be remembered that the parents, by their agreement, committed their child to the discomfort of the operation and separation from the family: it is not surprising that they show extreme interest in its outcome.

The aim of post-operative treatment

The aim of post-operative treatment is to enable the child to make the best use of the increased potential created by surgery. The aim is not to increase function, unless that was the aim of surgery. The surgical aim might be cosmetic, in which case increasing function is not post-operative treatment but a separate aim of treatment, running parallel to the post-operative aim, which would be to improve appearance.

This may appear to be splitting hairs, and of course in a sense it is, but, unless the aims are clearly seen it is easy for the therapist to lose sight of the purpose of the treatment.

To carry out effective post-operative treatment, it is essential to establish approximately:

(1) The time it takes after an operation for the benefit to become evident.

(2) For how much of that time he can benefit from intensive physiotherapy, and continued 'casual' physical management.

(3) When we can stop treatment and let the child get on with his life, or return to his pre-operative level of treatment.

There is a danger of post-operative treatment being regarded as *any* treatment which occurs after an operation. It is not: it is the treatment aimed at maximizing the aims of surgery.

(c) MANIPULATION AND STRAPPING

Some congenital fixed deformities respond to corrective manipulation: stretching the tight structures. These procedures need to be carried out early, frequently and fully. In some instances a well-corrected position can be maintained over a longer period by firm strapping after each manipulation (*Figure 16*). Manipulation can usually be taught to the parents; but particular care is necessary if the child has a sensory loss over the area.

(d) FRACTURES

The treatment of fractures has three consecutive aims:

(1) Reduction.

(2) Immobilization.

(3) Rehabilitation.

Of these, the first two are not the concern of the physiotherapist, (but *see* 'spontaneous fractures', p. 67) and the last has little relevance with children. Adams (17), who enthusiastically advocates physiotherapy for adult fracture patients, states 'so far as children are concerned supervised exercises are relatively unimportant and in most cases the child may safely be left to his own endeavours, aided when necessary by encouragement from the parents, who should always be fully informed of the programme of treatment and the likely course of events'.

We agree, but are pleased that some surgeons find it convenient to use the physiotherapy department to keep the patients and parents informed. Occasionally physiotherapy has a specific role. After long immobilization in bed walking training may be necessary,

80

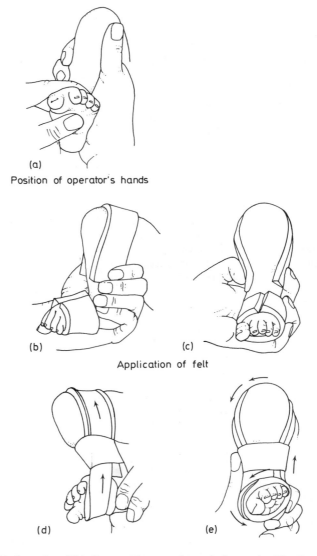

(a)

Position of operator's hands

(b)

(c)

Application of felt

(d)

(e)

Figure 16. Strapping. (This diagram illustrates the method as used at The Hospital for Sick Children 1967)

usually with some support in the first instance. A very few lessons at each stage will almost certainly suffice with all but the most timid child.

(e) MOBILIZATION OF JOINTS

Disease, trauma or spontaneous haemorrhage can each be the cause of limitation in joint range. In general terms physical treatment either needs to be carried out with great care or is unnecessary: a child's joint is either in danger from injudicious movement or able to be subjected to normal activities. Examples of the first category are mobilization after an acute episode of Still's disease or intra-articular haemorrhage from haemophilia. In the second category are found nearly all in which the cause was prolonged immobilization or trauma.

A programme of mobilization will include muscle re-education, because to prevent instability adequate muscle control must accompany any increase in joint range.

Some limitation of elbow movement is frequent after elbow joint dislocation or supracondylar fracture of the humerus. Occasionally this limitation can be severe. There are two common causes:

(1) Post-traumatic ossification of the haematoma.

(2) Malalignment.

Neither of these will respond beneficially to violent mobilization and gentle measures appear to have little effect. Provided the child uses the arm, the condition will either resolve to an acceptable state over a (long) period or it may require surgery. Traditionally such elbows do not belong in the physiotherapy department; however, this must be open to doubt since in a few patients treatment by an experienced physiotherapist produces a dramatic increase in joint range.

REFERENCES

(9) Daniels, L., Williams, M. and Worthington, C. (1956). *Muscle Testing—Techniques of Manual Examination*. Philadelphia: W. B. Saunders.

(10) Medical Research Council (1958). *Aids to the Investigation of Peripheral Nerve Injuries*. London: H.M. Stationery Office.

(11) Phelps, W. M. (1950). 'Etiology and diagnostic classification of cerebral palsy.' *Proceedings of the Cerebral Palsy Institute*. New York: Association for aid of Crippled Children, Inc.

(12) Crothers, B. and Paine, R. S. (1959). *The Natural History of Cerebral Palsy*. Cambridge, Mass.: Harvard University Press.

(13) Robson, P. (1970). 'Shuffling, hitching, scooting or sliding: some observations in 30 otherwise normal children.' *Dev. Med. Child. Neurol.,* **12**, 5. 608.
(14) Sharrard, W. J. W. (1971). *Paediatric Orthopaedics and Fractures.* Oxford and Edinburgh: Blackwell Scientific Publications.
(15) Finnie, N. R. (1974). *Handling the Young Cerebral Palsied Child at Home,* 2nd Edition. London: Heinemann Medical Books.
(16) Menelaus, M. B. (1971). *The Orthopaedic Management of Spina Bifida Cystica.* Edinburgh and London: Livingstone.
(17) Adams, J. C. (1958). *Outline of Fractures,* p.59. London: Livingstone.

CHAPTER 5

Systemic disorders

There are many diagnoses which, from a physical treatment point of view, do not fit neatly into any one category, e.g. rheumatoid arthritis, and in which the emphasis alters according to whether the condition is acute or chronic. There are other conditions which are properly systemic but in which physiotherapy is geared to one aspect only, an example is cystic fibrosis where the therapist's treatment is entirely concerned with respiration, although she needs a broader view of the condition so that she can talk intelligently with the parents. The conditions which would naturally fall into the above groups are diverse and are, therefore, discussed individually in Section II.

CHAPTER 6

Skin disorders

Physiotherapy in the treatment of skin conditions has enjoyed peaks of popularity over the years. Ultra-violet light is the medium most used (*see* Electrotherapy, Appendix 7). In many cases its use has been superseded; but it still has a contribution to make in some situations, e.g. in the treatment of indolent ulcers, and this is discussed in Section II.

Some exercises related to movement development

It is both impractical and outside the scope of this book to give a detailed description of exercises. The illustrations that follow are intended to do no more than highlight a few aspects of treatment and with brief descriptions summarize the principles involved.

Creeping (Crawling) (*Figure 17*)

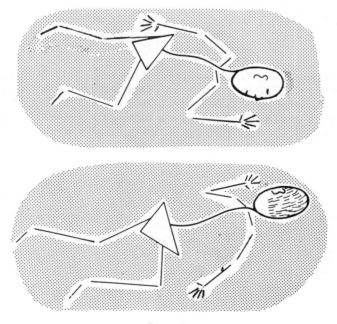

Figure 17

There is confusion about the terms creeping and crawling. To the authors creeping means that the body is on the ground, whilst in crawling it is supported on hands and knees. We realize that we may be at odds with many people, but, since we find that this is what the parents of our patients understand, it is the language we continue to use.

Symmetrical and asymmetrical limb movements, which mimic creeping, can be elicited in a number of ways. These movements are sometimes used because of their place in the so called 'ontogeny/ phylogeny' of movement. This seems to be of doubtful importance. They are included here from a quite different motive. In early treatment they are a useful means of producing a variety of total body movements, so that the infant is not experiencing one or two stereotyped postures only.

Lying prone (*Figures 18 and 19*)

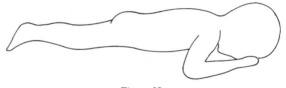

Figure 18

An infant may be helpless in prone if left on his own. With manual support or a prone ramp he can experience head extension and shoulder/shoulder girdle support. It is a good position in which to learn early head control, head turning for vision, hearing and for play.

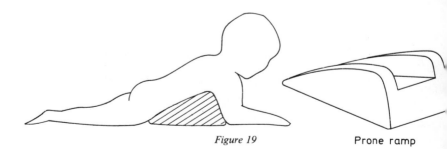

Figure 19   Prone ramp

Supine (*Figure 20*)

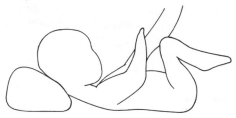

Figure 20

Playing in flexion. Note the head in the mid-line and in flexion.

Rolling (*Figure 21*)

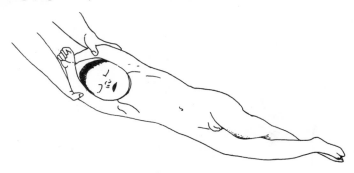

Figure 21

A method of giving the child an experience of co-ordinated total body movement to achieve an end, which by including trunk rotation helps break away from mass patterning.

Crawl position (*Figure 22*)

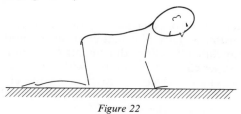

Figure 22

A difficult position for many children with a movement disorder as it combines so much flexion of the legs (without flexor spasm) and yet needs powerful and controlled extension of the arms. It is often useful to help develop elbow extension in movement-retarded children.

Getting up to standing (*Figure 23*)

Many children who have difficulty in getting up to standing use their arms to do most of the work. Normal children seldom use their arms *to pull* themselves up to standing or to take weight when on their feet: their arms are for stability, not weight-bearing.

One way of getting to standing is through half kneeling, pushing upwards and forwards (*Figure 23.*)

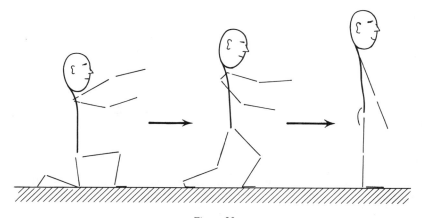

Figure 23

Another method is from a crouch position (*Figure 24*). For many children extension activity is a matter of all or nothing and this makes standing difficult as fine adjustments to maintain balance are impossible. Experience of standing without this uncontrolled extensor effort can be given by introducing the child's extensor activity from a flexed to a more extended position. It is essential that he is made to come upwards and forwards.

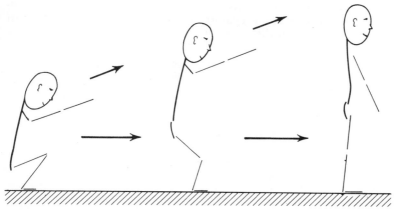

Figure 24

Standing (*Figure 24*)

Standing means taking the weight through the feet—not being poised upright in a baby-walker ('perambulating nappy') or suspended in a bouncer ('vertical playpen'). Both of these show a child how *not* to stand. It is essential that he should realize that his feet are his base and that his body has to be supported on them and balanced over them. In a bouncer or a walker his trunk becomes his base and so his legs can be drawn up from the floor without disturbing his stability, *see Figure 12*, page 45.

Early correct standing (from about 10 months) is thought to increase hip joint stability and we recommend that the child be placed in a standing position whenever there is reason for believing that spontaneous standing will be seriously delayed. Where there is asymmetric involvement we take greater care to ensure that both feet are taking weight. The child is supported as low down as possible (on the body or lower limbs) and can then practise balancing.

Walk standing (*Figure 25*)

Normal walking requires the leading leg to bear weight while the hip is slightly externally rotated and abducted. This is difficult for most cerebral palsy children, for whom extension of the hips and knees is combined with internal rotation and adduction. Practice in a correct walk-standing position is useful (particularly after most lower limb orthopaedic surgery).

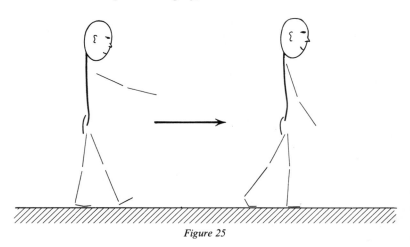

Figure 25

Manipulation (*Figures 26, 27 and 28*)

Infants who cannot explore on their own need a variety of experience brought to them. Their toys should have different shapes, weight, colours and textures. The child should be helped to play with both hands and watch what they are doing. This help can start early:

Figure 26

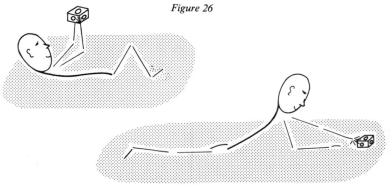

The infant can experience sound in relation to vision, using toys which make a noise.

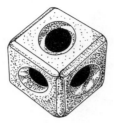

Figure 27

Play with their own body is important, experiencing that when (say) their hands touch their feet, their feet feel their hands.

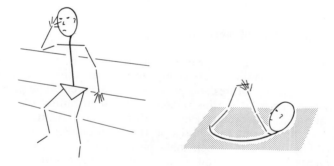

Figure 28

APPENDIX 2

Some of the factors affecting primitive and pathological posture and movement

(1) Mass patterning of movement

In nearly all hypertonic movement disorders of the CNS, there is a tendency for certain muscle groups to work together and so produce stereotyped postures and patterns of movement. The position adopted at one joint is thus related to the distribution of muscle 'tone' about all other joints. Physiotherapists take advantage of this effect and, by altering the child's posture, can influence movement ability. The degree to which mass patterning influences a child's movements is one indication of the severity of the disorder.

These mass movements are commonly divided into flexion and extension patterns: this division is convenient, provided it is remembered that it is an artifical classification. The patterns are well described in the literature, but it is worth examining one to show the difficulties it can create. There is basically one extension pattern seen in the legs: extension (with adduction and internal rotation) at the hip, extended knee and plantarflexed ankle. Producing any one of these movments makes the others more likely to occur. In normal adult walking this combination of movements is only required at push-off, which is about five per cent of the gait cycle. For the remaining time there is a mixture of flexion and extension at these joints. It is not surprising that children, whose movements are dominated by mass patterning, find normal walking difficult, and so resort to their own method.

(2) Asymmetric tonic neck response (ATNR)* *(Figure 29)*

This response is elicited by rotation of the head to one side. The response may be unilateral; sometimes only one side of the body *responds*: at others rotation to one side only will *produce* a response.

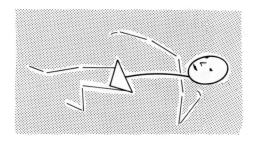

Figure 29. Rotation of the head to one side produces extension of the 'face-side' limbs and flexion of the 'occipital-side' limbs

The response, which is frequently apparent only when the child is supine or when he turns his head himself, is extension of the limbs on the face side, and flexion of the limbs on the 'occipital' side. The trunk response is variable but flexion to the occipital side is usual.

(3) Symmetrical tonic neck response (STNR) *(Figure 30)*

Like the ATNR this is a variable response. Extension of the head elicits extension of the arms and flexion of the legs. Flexion of the head produces flexion of the arms and extension of the legs. The STNR is most apparent when a brain-damaged child attempts a crawl position.

---

* Responses (2) to (6) are often called reflexes, but the authors prefer 'responses': they are seldom so invariable as the first term implies.

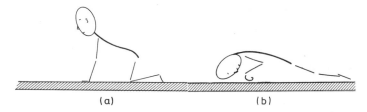

(a)   (b)

Figure 30. (a) Extension of the neck produces extension of the arms and flexion of the legs. (b) Flexion of the neck produces flexion of the arms and extension of the legs

(4) Tonic labyrinthine response (TLR)

The movement development of hypertonic infants may be influenced greatly by the position of the head relative to the horizontal plane. The TLR affects the distribution of muscle tone throughout the body. For simplicity it can be considered that a supine position favours extensor tone and prone favours flexor tone. Thus in many respects this response reinforces the effect of gravity.

(5) Positive supporting reaction or the extensor thrust response

Although experimentally these are two distinct reflexes, in the brain-injured child it is difficult to decide whether one or both are the culprits: it is also immaterial. In effect, weight bearing on the feet produces a massive extension of the legs which, although it mimics standing, tends to oppose the development of useful standing. It is because of this response that physiotherapists so abhor baby bouncers ('vertical pláypens') for children with cerebral palsy and some other disorders.

(6) Moro or startle response

The Moro response is normal during a baby's early months, after which it is superseded by more sophisticated movements. The brain-injured child often retains this primitive response to *any* excessive stimulus throughout his life. By its nature it occurs at the most inconvenient moments: in those situations when the correct response (balance, protection, grasp) is essential.

(7) Associated or overflow movements

Alterations of posture which appear to be produced by an excitation of a nervous system with inadequate inhibition for the circumstance. Such movements (or postures) are seen in the normal child and persist in certain circumstances throughout life. Normal associated movements differ from those seen in movement disorders: the former make the desired movement easier, whereas the latter interfere by distorting the background posture. An example is the change in arm position of the hemiplegic child from walking to running (*Figure 31*). The increased demands of running 'overflow' and the hemiplegic arm exaggerates its normal resting posture. A

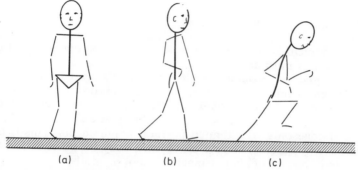

Figure 31. A child with right hemiplegia: (a) Standing, arm relaxed. (b) Walking, arm flexed. (c) Running, arm fully flexed

similar change of posture can be produced by getting the child to squeeze hard with the opposite hand, or indeed any other demanding action. These changes of posture can equally be induced by emotional tensions.

(8) Lack of movement experience

It is not known how great a part experience plays in the development of gross movement ability, for good arguments can be advanced on both sides. The answer may depend upon the point on the spectrum of movement complexity where we decide arbitrarily to use the word 'skilled'. Comparison with other situations leads us to consider that, in the normal mature locomotor system, movements are not either skilled or unskilled, but only more or less skilled. In the mature, but inadequate, locomotor system the level of skill—and therefore experience—required for a given movement could then be considered increased. One difficulty in discussing the importance of movement experience is that, although the normal locomotor system may overcome a lack of experience very quickly, we do not know whether this applies to the abnormal. Our experience indicates that in the abnormal specific practice is of far greater importance in movement development.

All of the foregoing factors will, in concert, produce an incorrect postural background for movement.

(9) Incorrect postural background

No movement is performed in isolation from the remainder of the body, which must adapt its posture to provide a secure base. The normal mature locomotor system fulfils this need by its almost unlimited combinations of movement and posture which are integrated by postural reflex mechanisms. The inadequate loco-motor system has limited possibilities of response available to it and so can cope only with limited postural requirements. This is one reason why certain discrete movements may be possible for the patient in one set of circumstances but not in another.

Balance and protective responses

Maintaining balance is a matter of keeping the line of gravity within the base. Therefore, the larger the base or the lower the centre of gravity, the greater is the stability. If the centre of gravity of the body is displaced there are three possible reactions:

(1) No active response—a free fall.

(2) Alteration of the relative position of the trunk and limbs to maintain the line of gravity within the base.

(3) Alteration of the base so that it is under the centre of gravity.

Altering the centre of gravity is called a balance response: altering the base is a protective response. Some of the 'parachute' reactions (18) are protective responses, although this depends on how they are elicited.

Balance responses

As an infant's ability for movement develops, so responses for balance emerge. The ability to balance in sitting does not imply a similar ability in crawling or standing. This unfolding of balance ability has lead to the examination of the age of appearance in various positions which are usually described for:

Prone—5 months

Supine—7 months

Sitting—7 to 8 months

Crawling—8 to 12 months

Standing—12 to 21 months

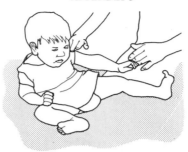

Figure 32. The balance response to sideways displacement in sitting maintains the centre of gravity over the buttocks

When the response is present in prone a similar response can usually be elicited in oblique suspension (*Figure 33*) (19).

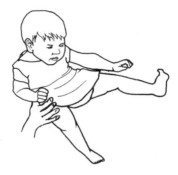

Figure 33. The response to oblique suspension commonly present by the age of 6 months

This time-table is of obvious use in a developmental examination, but like all classification it can be misleading. There are both neurological and environmental factors in this development, and what is crudely divided into five categories is in reality a continuously developing ability. An infant does not learn to balance in sitting *at a certain age*: he is first able to balance in sitting with a little support, then less support, and finally in increasingly adverse circumstances. So it is hard to say precisely when 'the balance reaction in sitting' has appeared.

Similarly (and perhaps more obviously) we are all aware of the large time lag between the appearance of the balance reaction in standing and the ability to stand on one leg, or on tip-toe on one leg, and few of us ever achieve what might be called a 'Blondin Response'!*

Protective Responses

Whether or not these reactions occur in lying must be a matter of definition, but they are usually considered to appear first in sitting. On being displaced suddenly and sufficiently to one side the infant's arm will extend and act as a prop, thus enlarging his base. The

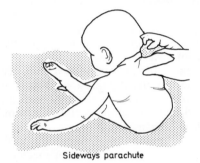

Sideways parachute

Figure 34. The protective response to sideways displacement in sitting moves the base under the displaced centre of gravity

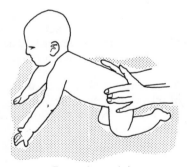

Forward parachute

Figure 35. The protective response to forward displacement in kneeling moves the base forwards under the displaced centre of gravity

* Charles Blondin (1824–1897), who walked a tight-rope across Niagara Falls.

classification is based on the ability to react to displacement in different directions and is usually tested in sitting or kneeling.

Sideways—6 months (*Figure 34*)

Forwards—7 months (*Figure 35*)

Like the balance reaction these responses merge imperceptively as the infant's general movement ability and experience increase and are effective in more and more elaborate positions and circumstances.

Propping on one upper limb already placed at his side is not necessarily a protective response, which to be fully performed requires the active movement into the propping position as part of the response to displacement. Many movement-handicapped children can prop and yet cannot respond to displacement because the correct response is superseded by a Moro reflex, a mass flexion of the arm, or disinterest.

Protective, or base shifting, responses also occur in the lower limbs, although they are usually not given this name. Displacement sideways, backwards or forwards can be compensated by taking a step in the appropriate direction. Walking is sometimes described as a volitional use of this mechanism.

There appears to be some undefined, but definite, connection between the delayed use of base altering mechanisms and mental retardation (*see* page 57).

The balance and protective responses are used to teach different types of movement because:

(1) Neither reaction necessarily requires the child's active co-operation, so that an involuntary, but active, treatment is possible.

(2) The movements of a balance reaction and a protective reaction are opposed to each other and so a wide range of movements can be elicited.

(3) The stimulus required to elicit each of them is different, so that some degree of selection is possible.

(4) More than any other discrete reactions they are the corner-stone of mature movement ability.

REFERENCES

(18) Milani-Comparetti, A., and Gidoni, E. A. (1967). 'Routine developmental examination in normal and retarded Children.' *Dev. Med. Child. Neurol.,* **9** (5). 631.

(19) Peiper, A. (1963). *Cerebral function in infancy and childhood.'* International Behavioural Sciences Series. (Ed. by J. Wortis), pp.180–190. New York: Consultants Bureau.

A rationale for the early treatment of movement disorders or delay

A case against the treatment of many movement disorders caused by disorganization of the higher centres can be summed up by three statements:

(1) A deficiency of the central nervous system is responsible for the disorder.

(2) Physical treatment cannot reduce this deficit.

(3) Therefore physical treatment cannot alter the disorder.

This argument is as unassailable as it is irrelevant. Physiotherapists need not refute it, because the case can be put another way:

(1) A defect of the central nervous system is responsible for the disorder.

(2) This will prevent the child functioning above a certain level of competence.

(3) Without help, will he *inevitably* function up to that level?

We contend that he is unlikely to do so. In fact we would go further and suggest that in many disorders and circumstances he certainly will not. The movement limitation and deformity which is often taken to be the *inevitable* outcome of brain damage is inevitable only if the child is subjected to an ordinary environment. To have a movement or postural deficit is (by implied definition) to be unable to cope with an ordinary environment which, by restricting activity, ensures the maximum opportunity of practising pathological movement responses and the minimum to experience the environment. Having accepted that the patient will inevitably have a motor disability, the physiotherapist aims to ensure that it is no greater than that directly attributable to the neural deficit.

This is shown diagrammatically in *Figure 36*. A limited movement potential leads to some sensory deprivation, incorrect movement

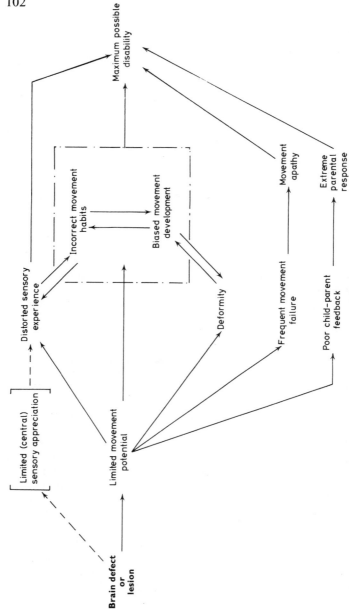

Figure 36. Cerebral palsy—the paths to maximum disability. Note: (i) different treatment methods concentrate their attention on different areas of this diagram; (ii) treatment aims will vary with many factors, such as disability or age

habits and (usually) deformities. The incorrect movement habits, which reinforce the limited movement potential, themselves increase both the sensory deprivation and the deformity.

Each of these in its turn makes correct movement more difficult and so reinforces the incorrect habits, all of these together make achievement difficult and so reduce the motivation to move. This diagram highlights the basic aims of treatment, and individual physiotherapists and treatment methods place different emphasis upon them.

Incorrect movement habits

As extensor ability develops during first few weeks of life; a baby placed in prone lifts his head so making it easier to free his arms. His arms also move away from the neonatal flexor-dominated posture and support his shoulders off the ground. This unfolding of the body as it explores its new environment—gravity—is sometimes attributed to reflex action of the most simple kind and there is no doubt this plays a part; but it appears unlikely that the intact CNS, even in its immature state, is quite so elementary that all its achievements can be ascribed to the inter-action of a series of chain reflexes (19). Certainly it is interesting to see how well an infant with Klippel–Feil syndrome may carry out the (anatomically possible) movements of some responses, without the supposedly necessary starting link to these 'chains'. However, the infant with an imperfect locomotor system is more limited, and here reflexes can and do play a greater part in movement: although many of the reported 'reflexes' are little more than responses in most instances.

For whatever reason, the infant lying prone should attempt to lift his head, but if pathological reflex activity maintains a flexor dominance in this position he will be unable to do so. With a little physical help he might overcome that dominance and so experience extension of his neck (and later support on his arms); but on his own he cannot do so but learns that 'prone equals flexion' or rather 'prone equals not-extension'. In fact head movement may be so difficult in prone that his mother keeps him on his back for fear of his suffocating.

Placed on his back he should be able to learn to move and to resist gravity, but not with his head, because even a normal infant cannot do that for several months. Upper and lower limbs are in neonatal flexion (fetal) postures which, in supine, are gravity resisting. However, the reflex flexor bias of prone is often replaced by extension in supine and the handicapped infant, once again finds both gravity and his central nervous system combining to oppose his attempts to move. Being safe on his back he is likely to be left in this position and has the maximum opportunity to learn that 'supine equals extension' or 'not-flexion'.

These two examples represent many situations facing the child throughout his movement development. There seems good clinical evidence to suggest that, by confronting such infants with an ordinary environment, we succeed only in teaching them how to perfect their disability.

Biased movement development

The locomotor developmental sequence is often written of as though it were a journey on a single-track railway: it is assumed that a child *must* pass through crawling before arriving at standing. Of course, it is accepted that there may be delays, but it is assumed that there is only one route. The fact that this is demonstrably untrue (13) appears not to concern the single-track lobby, who at the most will allow the use of detours around some of the stations.

The increasing complexity of definitive postural responses (which normally appear between the fifth and twelfth months of life) runs parallel to a more sophisticated ability to cope with the environment. As new intrinsic abilities appear (in the main, balance and protective responses, *see* Appendix 3) they will be utilized by a system exploring its own greater movement ability and efficiency. It should not be surprising that an infant learns to achieve less demanding movements before the more demanding ones; nor that some of the movements seen earlier, such as trunk rotation, should later be part of the more complex abilities such as walking. Given the combination of the usual anatomical structure, an integrating and undamaged central nervous system and gravity acting with an unvarying force and direction, it would indeed be surprising if similarities of movement did not occur as the locomotor system overcomes its environment. Thus locomotor development is *consequent upon* a normal CNS and it should not be assumed that this apparently logical and sequential development necessarily applies to the abnormal. There appears to be no simple cause–effect relationship between the acquisition of a response and its application to a function, although there is, of necessity, a strong affinity between the two.

The usual locomotor developmental sequence represents the most efficient locomotor activities for a 'normal' infant; we should expect a different sequence wherever there is abnormality either of the central nervous system or of the anatomical structure—and this is what we find*. It cannot follow that educating a child to move in the normal sequence will make him move more normally (any more than training a normal child in abnormal sequences will make him abnormal). It may, however, succeed in making him *less* efficient than he could be: it depends on how severely handicapped he is in relation to that movement. An essential part of assessment is deciding which movement sequences will be to his overall advantage.

A simple example of this can be seen in the development of an infant of average intelligence, good vision etc., but with infantile hemiplegia. He is unlikely to crawl, because his affected arm cannot support him, but will walk, usually not later than late normal. Many hemiplegic infants replace this intermediate locomotor stage by hitching (or shuffling). The crawl *position* may be useful as an exercise to widen general movement experience and more particularly to help gain extension of the flexed arm. However, to prevent a child from getting to standing and walking because he still cannot crawl is obviously absurd; yet the authors have seen this being done in the name of therapy.

Distorted sensory experience

Occasionally a patient gives us a brief insight of a particular misconception he holds of himself or his environment: perhaps a lack of understanding of shape, either kinesthetic or visual, a lack of body image or of some other fundamental concept. We can never *know* how normal perception varies from that of a patient with a congenital movement disability, but the available evidence suggests that it does. Deprived of free movement, the environment probably appears very different.

The inability to reach for a toy deprives the child of the proprioception of the movement: how far away the toy is, the eye–hand co-ordination, the size, texture, shape and weight of the toy, and much more besides. Immobility precludes experience of how large a bed or room is, or that the window is not a picture. Without such

* Or for that matter alterations of gravity or the medium in which we move. Television from the moon has shown how alteration of these factors radically changes 'normal' movement.

information the brain is unable to respond correctly to the environment. Treatment cannot fully replace such a deficit, but by ensuring that a wide range of experience, kinesthetic, tactile, thermal, visual etc. is brought to the child some improvement in appreciation of his body and his surroundings can be anticipated. It is an important aspect of physical treatment.

Deformity

A continuous imbalance of forces about a joint will inevitably lead to some distortion of the bones and soft tissues involved. The imbalance need not be caused by overactivity of one muscle group in relation to another: gravity will do the job quite as well.

Hypotonic children—more frequently the severely retarded— lie with their hips and knees in flexion. The unopposed pull of

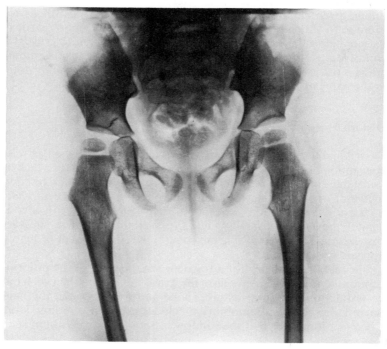

(a

Figure 37. Gradual dislocation of the hip over a five year period: a child with cerebral palsy. (a) Aged 4 years

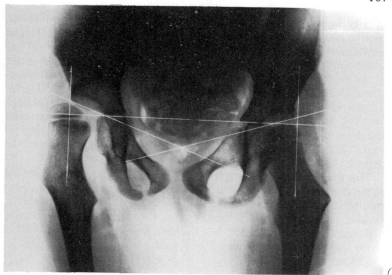

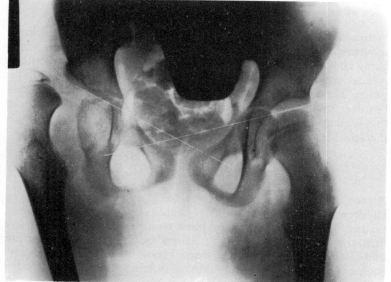

Figure 37. Gradual dislocation of the hip over a five year period: a child with cerebral palsy. (b) Aged 6 years. (c) Aged 9 years

gravity keeps their legs in full external rotation and abduction, with consequent structural deformity of the femoral neck and sometimes anterior subluxation of the hips. Hypertonicity in the lower limbs favours adduction, internal rotation of the lower limbs at the hips leading to the opposite deformity of femoral neck anteversion. Subluxation or dislocation is again possible, but bilateral dislocation is seldom seen in the hypertonic group—perhaps because such serious involvement implies a strong asymmetric tonic neck response. These dislocations develop over a period of years (*Figure 37 a, b and c*) and there is good clinical evidence to believe that many of them are preventable.

The fixed deformities are usually referred to as 'contractures', a name derived from adult orthopaedics, but there is little to support its use in this instance. More likely these deformities represent a lack of growth of certain muscles due to an imbalance of forces. This may appear semantics, but because lack of growth is different from contracture it requires different treatment. This point is discussed elsewhere (p. 46).

Lack of movement success

With every attempt at movement frustrated, particularly accurate movements which are the most purposeful, it is not surprising that many children give up making the effort. Such continuous ineffectiveness must be intolerable to anyone with even moderate intelligence. They *must* be given the opportunity to experience success, however small, and contriving circumstances in which to achieve this is an important part of what the physiotherapist does. Physiotherapists instil this aim into those looking after these children.

THE SEVERELY MENTALLY RETARDED CHILD

Although a reference has already been made in this chapter to children with movement delay caused by mental retardation, further brief consideration of these children is necessary. Severe mental subnormality appears to bring about movement retardation and distortion in a number of ways. Inevitably any simple scheme, such as *Figure 38*, is open to addition or amendment; it is included to highlight two points: (*a*) there is more than one reason for physical treatment; (*b*) some of the aims of treatment are the same for both mental subnormality and locomotor disorder.

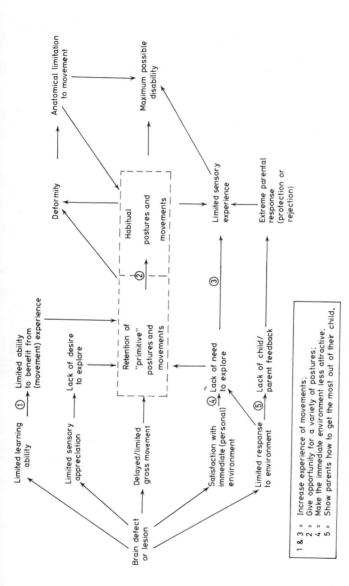

Figure 38. *The severely mentally retarded child: The paths to maximum disability and where physiotherapy can interrupt them. 1 and 3=increase experience of movements; 2=give opportunity for a variety of postures; 4=make the immediate environment less attractive; 5=show parents how to get the most out of their child*

REFERENCES

(13) Robson, P. (1970). 'Shuffling, hitching, scooting or sliding: some observations on 30 otherwise normal children.' *Dev. Med. Child. Neurol;* **12** (5) 608.
(19) Peiper, A. (1963). *Cerebral function in infancy and childhood.* International Behavioural Sciences Series. (Ed. by J. Wortis), pp. 180–190. New York: Consultants Bureau.

Some methods of physical support

External support may be needed for several reasons.
(1) To maintain balance.
(2) For protection.
(3) For rest.
(4) To maintain or improve skeletal alignment—perhaps to supplement inadequate or unbalanced muscle action.

In all instances the prescriber should bear in mind whether the aim is to replace a function and/or to re-educate a function.

Balance

Head. A variety of devices have been made to help head control in sitting. They range from rigid structures attached to a chair which clamp the head in one position or allow some rotation; through those which suspend the head with springs so that the child can learn to appeciate better head control; to simple pads either side of the head fixed to the chair back.

Trunk. Simple straps or harness are often used for trunk stability in sitting. Where education of function is important the harness may be fitted firmly around the child, but loosely to the chair so as to allow a certain amount of movement within the child's ability.

Sometimes it is more convenient and practical to use a tray with a cut-out for the body to act as a trunk support as well as a working surface. This is likely to be more supportive than educational.

Whole body in standing. Standing requires a secure base and good balance. A few (usually hypotonic) children can be helped to stand and walk by fitting below knee outside irons and inside 'T' straps to improve ankle/foot stability: boots alone may help. When fitted for this reason such support seldom needs retaining for more than a few months after walking has been achieved. The more usual solution to balance difficulties is to give the child some means of support higher up: either reducing the balance problem (suspending him in a full harness in a frame) or transferring the responsibility to his arms and enlarging his effective base. Examples of this latter method are parallel bars, various walking aids, both with skids or wheels, quadrapods, tripods, crutches or walking sticks (*Figure 39*). The decision as to which is best for a child at a particular stage of his treatment or motor development can best be made by the physiotherapist, as many factors are involved in the decision.

Protection

Examples of this use of support are seen in bracing for ununited fracture and splinting to prevent the over-stretching of denervated muscles.

Rest

In some conditions relaxation of all or part of the body is essential, either to reduce pain or aid recovery. This is made easier if the responsibility for combating gravity can be passed from the child's muscles to some external support, such as plaster of paris or thermoplastic shells, plastic foam pads, sand bags or pillows.

Skeletal alignment

The aims of treatment are: (*a*) to prevent or correct structural or fixed deformity; and (*b*) to improve function.
    These will be discussed together as they so often overlap.

Upper limbs

A wide range of supports have been used on the arms, particularly devices for assisting or maintaining wrist dorsiflexion, thumb

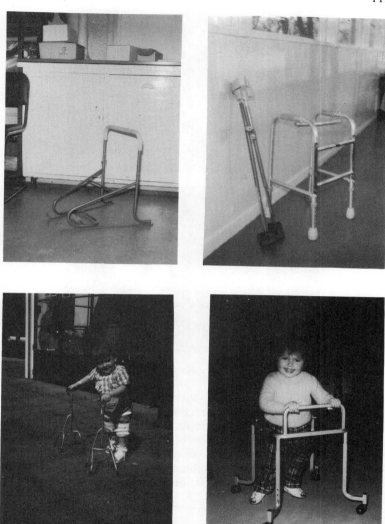

Figure 39. A selection of walking aids. Each appliance has advantages over the others in certain circumstances. A physiotherapist knows which is the best for the patient (contd. on p.114)

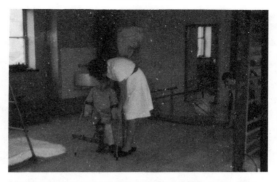

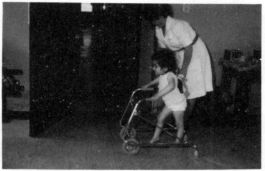

Figure 39 contd.

abduction, elbow flexion and total arm suspension (to replace shoulder and shoulder girdle function). The variety of apparatus is as much a reflection of the arm's wide range of activities (and therefore possible disabilities) as of the difficulties of designing a device capable of more than one or two functions. The simplest support is probably the infant's thumb abduction splint (*Figure 40*): an example of the more elaborate devices is shown in *Figure 41*.

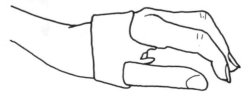

Figure 40. Thumb abduction splint

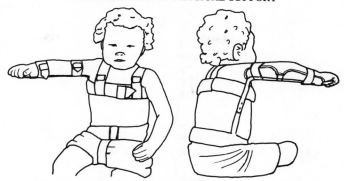

Figure 41. A splint to maintain abduction at the shoulder joint

Trunk

The maintenance and development of vertical alignment is a complex subject well beyond the scope of this book. However external methods of inducing better lateral alignment have two basic means: three point pressure (*Figure 42a*) and distraction (*Figure 42b*).

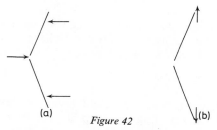

Figure 42

Three point pressure in its simplest form relies on gravity for two of the points and a support for the third (*Figure 43*).

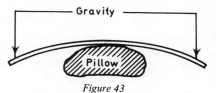

Figure 43

In a chair many children who do not need more definite correction can be supported by the relative position of the restraining straps and side supports (*Figure 44*).

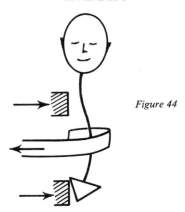

Figure 44

The use of any more firmly corrective methods is a matter for the orthopaedic department and (when prescribed) the physiotherapist's function is confined to exercises (*see* p. 179) and, intermittently, to checking the fit of the brace.

Distraction.   This method applies mainly to the Milwaukee type brace (which combines distraction with three point pressure) and its more recent modifications.

A reduction of the compressive force (but without distraction) occurs when the spine is taken away from the vertical: tilting a chair back (say) 20 degrees will reduce some of the deforming forces.

Lower limbs

Footwear.   On a pre-walking child boots or shoes protect the socks and feet when crawling and keep the feet warm. The function is different from that of ambulant footwear and the design should reflect this difference. When walking, feet still need warmth and protection, but protection from a different direction (the underside) and from greater forces which are now applied with at least body weight. This latter requirement demands a more rigid structure and so correct fitting is of greater importance. However, the current mystique surrounding children's shoes (20) mimics dogma whilst masking commonsense. In warm climates footwear need only protect the underside of the feet; when cold, footwear should also keep the feet warm. A 'shoe' should not compress a foot, should allow for growth and yet not permit the sole or heel to move relative to the foot. In some disorders affecting feet the child's toes cannot be prevented from being flexed unless the upper can be undone right to the toe of the boot. This design is available commercially and, together with an increasing range of more suitable boots and shoes, reduces the need for surgical footwear. Nevertheless a few children will require individually made boots or shoes although this requirement is unsuitable practically and economically for growing children.

Footwear for bracing. Most bracing of the lower limbs has a distal anchoring point in the boot or shoe. There is an obvious, and yet often neglected, necessity for the footwear (i) to fit correctly, (ii) to be made to withstand the new forces being applied to it and (iii) to transmit them to the foot. The key to lower limb bracing is the concept of three point pressure mentioned above.

Foot and ankle. Below knee bracing is used to control varus, valgus, equinus or calcaneus. For varus or valgus control a single iron is usually enough and is combined with a 'T' strap which acts as the third force (*Figure 45*).

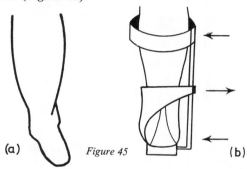

(a)   *Figure 45*   (b)

Equinus or calcaneus usually requires a double iron (caliper) and 'stops' to prevent equinus or calcaneus or both. Where the range of

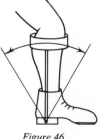

Figure 46

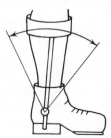

Figure 47

ankle movement is small the anchoring point of the brace can also be the axis of the hinge (heel spur fixing, *Figure 46*), but if much movement is required (and usually with any form of spring assistance for dorsiflexion) a separate hinge is fitted at ankle joint level (*Figure 47*) and the heel mounting is rigid.

Knee. Knee extension is usually maintained by extending the below knee type caliper* over the knee to the thigh (*Figure 48*). The three pressure points are: (1) the posterior thigh cuff; (2) the back of the shoe; and (3) the knee pad.

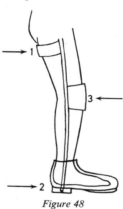

Figure 48

There may be hinges at the knee to make sitting easier: these are locked for standing. Knee hyperextension can be prevented by a similar hinged brace (without locks) which has limited knee extension and a pad in the popliteal fossa.

Weight relieving calipers appear similar to those shown above but are made so that the upper cuff bears on the ischial tuberosity. In this way part of the patient's weight is borne by the caliper and not by the lower limb (*Figure 49*).

Hip. There are two reasons for extending a brace up over the hips: (*a*) to control the lower limbs in relation to each other; and (*b*) to control the lower limbs in relation to the trunk.

A simple pelvic band connecting the two lower limb calipers can

---

* Originally *'Calliper'* compasses used for measuring the calibre of a bullet or piece of ordnance: presumably variant of 'calibre'—from Arab *Qualib*, mould for casting metal (from the *Oxford Dictionary of English Etymology*).

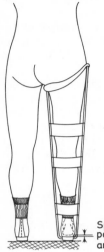

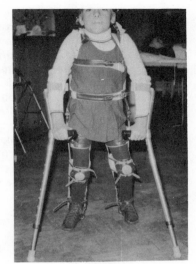

Space between
patient's heel
and boot

Figure 49.

Figure 50 (a)

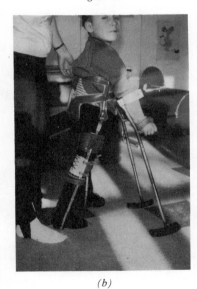

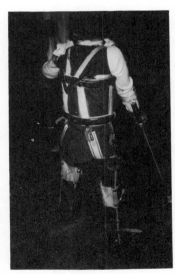

(b)

(c)

Figure 50

be used to limit hip adduction and abduction or external and internal rotation. It has little effect on flexion or extension.

If a caliper is fitted to one lower limb only, some control of hip abduction/adduction, external/internal rotation and flexion/extension can be obtained by making the pelvic band wider and moulding it closely to the pelvis.

Where the aim is bilateral control of flexion or extension, usually to prevent a collapse into flexion, then greater leverage is required and the pelvic band may have a thoracic band (*Figure 50a*) added above it. Alternatively it is replaced by a jacket or corset top.

The three point system tends to fail here as there is often insufficient support at the buttocks. This is usually overcome by a downwards extension of the pelvic band or a buttock sling (*Figure 50 (b) and (c)*).

REFERENCES

(20) Bleck, E. E. (1971). 'The shoeing of children: sham or science?' *Dev. Med. Child. Neurol.*, **13** (2), 188.

Sitting and chairs

Sitting deserves a description on its own because it is the most commonly used intermediate position between the relaxation of lying and the active postures of crawling or standing. It is the best position for so many activities and one in which many handicapped children are expected to live. There are six basic sitting positions (*Figure 51*).

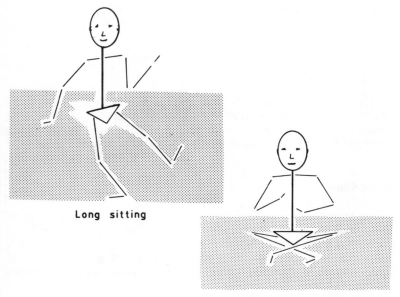

Long sitting

Cross legged sitting

Figure 51

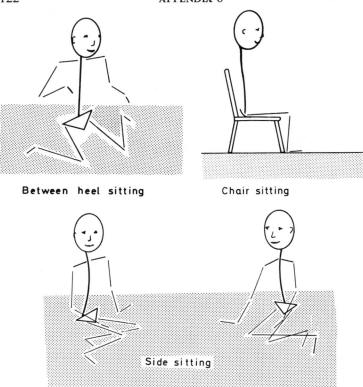

Between heel sitting　　　Chair sitting

Side sitting

Figure 51 (contd.)

Their common factor is that a large proportion of the body weight is taken through one or both ischial tuberosities. Providing comfortable and desirable sitting positions for handicapped children becomes very much easier when this is borne in mind.

Long sitting

Long sitting is the natural first sitting position for the majority of infants. By leaning forwards their centre of gravity is well inside a large triangular base. They are usually propped up in this position a couple of months before they can get up into it by themselves. It gives wide opportunities for seeing what is going on around them and for play, and allows them to practise their rapidly emerging gross motor skills (trunk equilibrium, arm propping, protective extension).

Their difficulty is remaining upright and not falling backwards when they overextend their spines. Poor motor control exaggerates this problem. Short/spastic hamstrings tend to throw the weight on to the sacrum rather than the ischial tuberosities. As a result the lower vertebrae are incorrectly aligned and compound the problem of trunk control (*Figure 52 a and b*): it is better for affected children to flex their knees slightly and so allow more hip flexion.

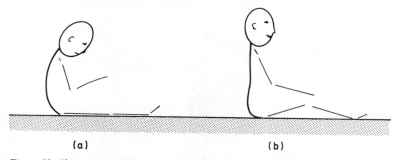

(a)   (b)

Figure 52. Short or spastic hamstring muscles may cause the child (a) to sit more on the sacrum than ischial tuberosities: (b) Semi-flexion at the knees relaxes the muscles and allows the hip flexion necessary for good trunk posture

Trunk control cannot be learnt without a secure base, so the infant needs his buttocks firmly supported. A corner seat (*Figure 53*) may help, but should be made for the particular child and be measured for height of back-rest, distance from crutch support to corner, height and size of tray. Unless the back-rest is also a head support it rarely needs padding: an infant is well padded by his napkins and clothes.

Cross-legged sitting

Cross-legged sitting is not a very useful position. The combination of a smaller base, together with the total flexion of the lower limbs makes this a difficult position for most handicapped children. It is misused by some physiotherapists for children who perpetually sit between heel—to get their hips away from an internally rotated

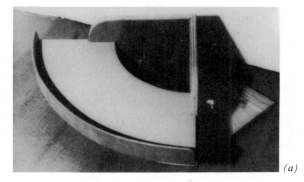

(a)

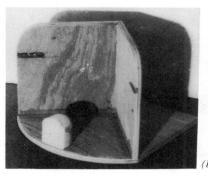

(b)

Figure 53. (a) A 'corner seat', like any appliance, must fit the child and his particular needs. The height of the backrest and tray (if fitted) and the position of the crutch block are of particular importance. The crutch block maintains the position of the pelvis and prevents the child adopting the posture shown in Figure 52 (a).
(b) The seat, with the tray removed showing the crutch block

position. Unfortunately it is these very children who find it hardest to do anything when placed cross-legged.

Between heel sitting

Between heel sitting is perhaps the *easiest* floor sitting position, particularly for a child (normal or abnormal) who has a good prone development. It is his natural resting posture from crawling and leads easily into upright kneeling and standing. The vertebral column is in the middle of a large base, the hamstrings are relaxed and so the pelvis is not tipped back, thereby upsetting trunk alignment. It is the classic sitting posture of the spastic diplegic and is blamed by many for their typical femoral neck deformities. In its favour, it is probably the best position for many children to learn correct trunk control and the relaxed hamstrings allow the development of the secondary lumbar curve.

Side sitting

Side sitting is a natural playing position for normal children. It gives a good base and allows the child to be right on top of whatever he is doing. For the handicapped child it has the disadvantage that it requires two good arms, one for support and the other for play. Its significance *as a posture* in handicapped children is almost entirely restricted to spastic hemiplegia: side sitting to the non-affected side being a favourite sitting and shuffling position. It is comfortable for them because it allows all their postural tendencies full reign—hip adduction/internal rotation, shortened hamstrings, trunk side flexion to the hemiplegic side and no effort by the hemiplegic arm.

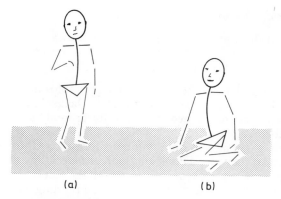

(a)　　　　　　　(b)

Figure 54. Side sitting and the management of hemiplegia (see text)

The position is used (but reversed) for therapy, since the child can play with his good hand, while (with help) learning an extension posture of his hemiplegic arm, trunk side flexion away from the involved side and hip external rotation (*Figure 54 a and b*).

Chair sitting

From the design of most children's chairs it might be thought that sitting means no more than being in a chair, regardless of the position adopted on it. It makes sitting *easier* for a normal child if a chair fits him reasonably well: it makes sitting *possible* for a handicapped child. What is meant by fit?

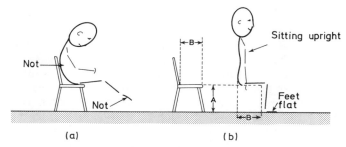

Figure 55. (a) Everybody is more comfortable in a chair that fits, but for a physically handicapped child it may make the difference between being able to sit to feed himself or write and being unable to sit at all. (b) The most important measurements are the length and height of the seat

Size (*Figure 55 a* and *b*)

Length.   If the seat is *too* long the child will lean back (*Figure 55a*) and probably slide his buttocks forwards: too short and he lacks the additional support of the full length of his thighs.

Height.   Too high and he cannot get support through his feet: too low and his hips are over-flexed and he lacks full length thigh support. The seat height need not be to the ground but to a foot-rest if more convenient.

There is a division of opinion about foot-rests: those in favour maintain that they give a constant floor surface, allow the feet to be fixed (if necessary), prevent thrusting with the feet from tipping the chair over backwards, and prevent the child pushing himself around backwards. Those against foot-rests maintain that it is easier to get on and off a chair without one and they *like* children to push themselves around backwards!

Back-rest height.   The back-rest should not support the head unless the child cannot control it well enough by himself, or unless (for some other reason) the chair has to be tipped backwards.

Back-rest slope. As a general rule the back-rest should be at an angle of approximately 100 degrees to the seat.

Support

Pelvis. Having a chair which fits for size may not be enough. The child may be too floppy, stiff or lack the necessary balance. The cardinal rule for supporting a child in a chair is to fix his pelvis in the correct position: that is, with his weight taken equally on both ischial tuberosities. If this is ignored all other measures will be in vain. It is surprising how often efforts are made to support a child with a strap around his chest without first controlling his pelvis.

Many infant's chairs allow the child to slide too far forward on the seat because the straps are fixed at the front of the seat (*Figure 56*).

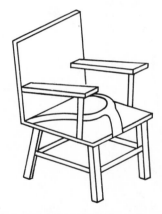

Figure 56. Most infant chairs have a 'groin strap' fitted incorrectly so the child can slide forward. See Figure 57 a, b and c

There are many ways (*Figure 57 a, b and c*) of holding the pelvis back, each of which has advantages and disadvantages, but if the child cannot maintain this position without aid then some means must be used, or all thought of correct sitting be abandoned.

Trunk. With the pelvis secure the child has the opportunity to learn trunk control: support may still be needed, but it is important to remember that the aims of this support may vary.

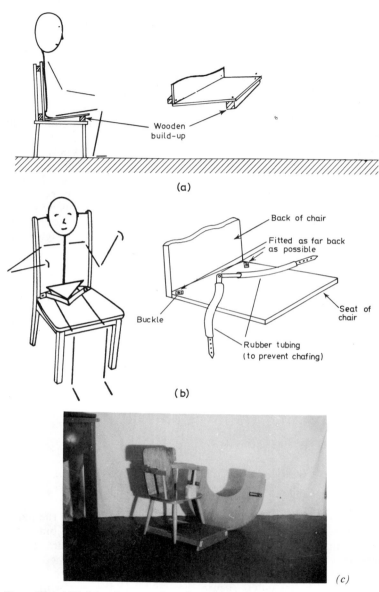

Figure 57. (a) Wedging the seat makes it harder for a child to slide forward. (b) 'Groin straps' should be fitted at least as far back as the groin. A trunk strap, if necessary, should be fitted separately and not as part of a groin strap. Combining the functions usually reduces the efficiency. (C) A crutch block is the most positive method of maintaining a correct sitting base. If it is fitted correctly, it is not uncomfortable for the child and is easier to use than straps

(1) If he has insufficient head control then the support to the trunk would be designed to supply a firm enough base for head control to be learnt.

(2) If he has fair to good head control then the trunk support must be just enough to give him the opportunity to learn trunk, control, i.e. there must be opportunity for free movement within and just beyond his range of ability.

(3) If he has little or no chance of learning better control, then it will be supportive only: (a) to give the best opportunity to function to his maximum; (b) to prevent deformity.

Feet. It is sometimes necessary to help the child to hold his feet in the correct position. Correctly placed, his feet can give good support to the rest of his body. At the same time he has the opportunity to appreciate postural control through his feet to his body, which may help his understanding their function in standing.

Wheelchairs (*Figures 58–63*) (21)

It is hard to overestimate the difficulties of designing a good wheelchair: so many of the requirements are mutually exclusive. When considering a wheelchair for a particular child it is pertinent to ask the following questions:

(1) Is it needed as a push-chair or as a self-propelled chair?

(2) Will it be used indoors, outdoors, or both?

(3) Will he be travelling in it to and from school, and using it at school?

(4) Will it have to be taken by car, on a bus or train?

(5) Where will it be kept at home?

All too often wheelchairs are issued without thought for the *other* users—the parents. A chair which suits the child may be far from what is needed by the parents, who may not realize their real need until closely questioned and shown the various alternatives available. Very often one chair alone cannot fulfil the needs: for

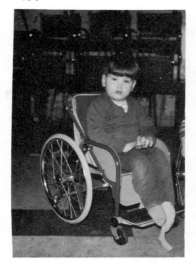

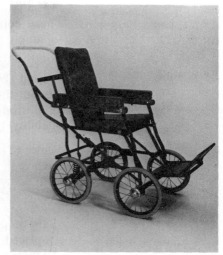

Figure 58. Yorkhill self-propelling chair for children aged approximately 2–6 years. (Reproduced by courtesy of The Department of Health and Social Security)

Figure 60. Push chair. (Reproduced by courtesy of The Department of Health and Social Security)

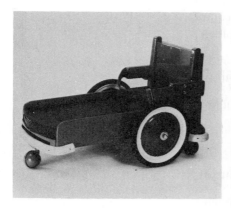

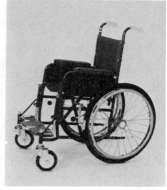

Figure 59. 'Chailey chariot' self-propelling floor level chair. (Reproduced by courtesy of The Department of Health and Social Security)

Figure 61. Self-propelling wheelchair. (Reproduced by courtesy of The Department of Health and Social Security)

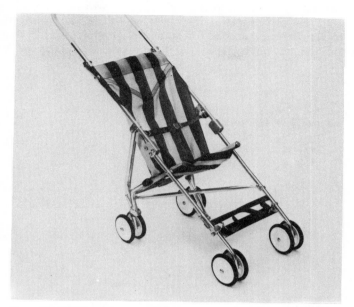

Figure 62. Baby buggy. (Reproduced by courtesy of Andrews Maclaren Ltd)

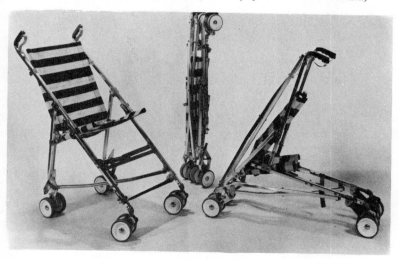

Figure 63. Major buggy. (Reproduced by courtesy of Andrews Maclaren Ltd)

instance one chair could give good support, provide a useful size tray and be self-propelled indoors, whilst another altogether lighter chair may be needed for going out shopping or for walks. The solution may not be cheap, but it is none the less correct for that.

REFERENCE

(21) Holt, K. S., Darcus, H. and Brand, H. L. (1972). 'Children's wheelchair clinic.' *Br. med. J.*, **4**, 651–655.

Electrotherapy

Discussion

Electrotherapy has comparatively little to offer paediatrics. Patient co-operation is essential for some treatments and so they may be ruled out by age. Others are so frightening to a small child and so uncomfortable that he is unable to endure an effective intensity: such treatments succeed only in encouraging a hatred of all association with hospital. This area of physiotherapy emphasizes the difference between treating children and adults perhaps more than any other, because the problem of discomfort is often introduced. An adult can appreciate that electrical stimulation aids muscle re-education. A child, however, is not able to accept a machine delivering regular pin-prick sensations—which are to him like injections—and will almost always be in tears long before an effective intensity is reached. Repeatedly subjecting a child to this experience cannot be justified. Similarly, he will not realize the necessity of reporting instantly any discomfort during a heat treatment (even adults need rigorous supervision). Applying deep heat, such as short-wave diathermy, to young children must be avoided whenever possible because of the dangers of burning.

There are exceptions, the most notable being electrical stimulation as an aid to diagnosis. This is usually an isolated incident and, if necessary, the child may be sedated. Very occasionally a child will accept and appear to benefit from some of the other treatments.

Muscle stimulation

Producing contractions by stimulating a muscle through its motor nerve requires short duration (1 msec) pulses, still often referred to as 'Faradic' stimulation. It is very seldom appropriate as a means of muscle re-education for children. However, low intensity faradic foot-baths for general stimulation of foot muscles can improve the local circulation and reduce local muscle spasm in some children with generalized movement disorders.

Where there is a peripheral nerve lesion, contractions can be produced by direct stimulation of the muscle and requires longer duration pulses (100 msec). There is a wide selection of pulse shapes and durations produced electronically, which are seldom used for children.

The diagnostic use of muscle and nerve stimulating currents has been referred to briefly in the discussion.

Infra-red radiation

The wave lengths used therapeutically are approximately between 64 000Å and 8000Å. Their effect is to produce heat when and where they are absorbed in the body. It is therefore natural that we should be concerned with their depth of penetration before absorption and for this reason they are usually divided into two groups:

Longer radiation (64 000Å to 16 000Å) which, being absorbed by water, cannot penetrate deeply.

Shorter radiation (16 000Å to 8000Å) certainly penetrates further, but to what depth in living tissue is not known.

Although these radiations do not have a large place in paediatric physiotherapy, they are sometimes used to promote relaxation of muscle spasm or before breathing training (with asthmatic children). As with all heat treatments, careful supervision is necessary.

Short-wave diathermy

This method of heating the deeper tissues is rarely used. Empirically determined subthermal doses sometimes appear to disperse swelling and haematoma, but it is interesting to note that in a department which undertakes approximately 40 000 children's treatments a year it was impossible to take part in a proposed trial of short-wave diathermy treatment as many months passed without any patients being referred.

Ultra-violet radiation

UVR has a consistent role in the treatment of children and it will be dealt with in greater detail.

The therapeutic effects of radiation between approximately 2000 and 4000Å units (the ultra-violet rays) are often overlooked. Their influence upon tissue function is so well known (sunburn, sun-tan and conjunctivitis) that it is always a surprise to physiotherapists when these rays are dismissed as part of 'heat lamps and all that stuff'. UVR has little more connection with infra-red rays than x-rays: it is a powerful (and therefore dangerous) band of radiation which is customarily divided by its two differing effects:

2000 to 2900Å (abiotic) (22): Exposure to these rays kills cells, so releasing histamine-like substances. Almost all these rays are absorbed by the cornified layer of the skin, but are often used on open wounds when greater penetration is possible. Uses: (*a*) sterilization of superficially infected wounds; and (*b*) promotion of healing by indirectly stimulating granulation.

2900 to 4000Å (biotic): these penetrate through the cornified layer of the skin, stimulating cell function, and can be used for: (*a*) accelerating healing of clean granulating areas; (*b*) accelerating epithelialization of superficial wounds; (*c*) increasing circulation of the superficial parts of the dermis.

General applications (for which the longer rays are more appropriate): currently little used. There were two main uses:

(1) It was common practice for 'debilitated' children to receive a course of general UVR to increase resistance to infection. The practice has fallen into disrepute, due to antibiotics and the abandonment of the 'old-fashioned' open arc generator. Although not the most up-to-date looking piece of apparatus, the open arc produced proportionately six times more of the longer wavelengths than the mercury arc. The advent of the newer fluorescent tube generators may gradually change this fashion again, for they are easier to use for general treatments and are said to produce no radiation below 2800Å.

(2) At one time radiation between 2700 and 2900Å was used for stimulation of vitamin D formation. The production of oral calciferol has effectively removed the need.

Dosage

The results of exposure to ultra-violet light are classified by the visible tissue response, and are described as degrees of erythema (E) ranging from 1°E to 4°E according to the following scale:

1°E: a faint pinkness which appears after approximately 12 hours and has completely faded within 24 hours.

2°E: pink response within 8 hours lasting up to two days and followed by fine desquamation.

3°E: red response within 8 hours, accompanied by discomfort for approximately two days, taking at least five days to fade completely, and followed by ready desquamation.

4°E: This dose produces a blister, is only used as a counter-irritant and rarely in children. Much larger doses, however, are frequently and usefully given to indolent open areas where skin response is irrelevant.

To summarize, UVR has one common use, for healing of ulcers, indolent wounds; and several possible uses with children: for treating acne, for treating psoriasis, for ultra-violet sensitivity testing.

REFERENCES

(22) Hausser, K. W. and Vahle, W. (1922). 'Die Abhängigkeit des Lichterythems und der Pigmentbildung von der Schwingungszahl (Wellenlänge) der Erregenden Strahlung.' *Strahlentherapie*, **13**, 41.

Hydrotherapy

In some circumstances, water has advantages over air as a medium surrounding the body. The properties used in hydrotherapy are:

(1) Greater density than air (and slightly greater than the body): it therefore eliminates gravity and replaces it by buoyancy. It also imparts an increased uniform pressure on the body surface, which appears to have a beneficial reflex effect, stabilizing postural control in some disorders of the central nervous system.

(2) Greater viscosity than air, which together with its greater density offers increased resistance to movement—particularly quick movement.

(3) Greater thermal capacity than air, so it is easier to control its temperature under treatment conditions.

Hydrotherapy for children can be divided into local and general.

Local uses

Hydrotherapy is used locally for (a) improving circulation; (b) re-educating muscle action; and (c) mobilizing joints.

There must still be a place for these treatments, which in the past played such a large part in the management of many chronic disorders of childhood. Their use has all but ceased and it is the changing pattern of disease, rather than any inefficiency of the treatment, which has brought this about. Consequently there are now few departments which can offer both the facilities and staff experienced in these treatments. Since it is the aim of this book to present treatments *available* to the doctor it would be unrealistic to elaborate on the rationale and methods. The situation is quite different from that of adults where, in certain disorders, hydrotherapy is a well established and valued means of treatment. The majority of physiotherapists working today can achieve better results by other means of treatment; whether these results are better than those obtained by their professional ancestors is uncertain.

General uses

Immersion in a particular river, spring, or hospital pool has a long and well documented attraction to man as a means of improving the 'inner-self', and has contrasted markedly with his changeable attitude to its effect on his exterior.

Despite the increasing sophistication of medicine and the public's attitude to disease, hydrotherapy retains a mystique, which serves only to hide its real therapeutic values. What then can pool therapy offer?

Exercise

General. Buoyancy allows many children to move more freely and experience the delight of movement. The psychological and physiological benefits of general exercise do not need elaboration.
Specific. The buoyancy and resistance to movement offered by water allow movements which would be impossible in air. Although the postural reactions required in water are different from those on land there are many similarities and they are also slower, which gives the child time to react and appreciate how to use his body.

Orientation

Observation suggests that many children with severe congenital or early acquired disorders of movement have difficulty in understanding space. They should be able to appreciate that three dimensional space exists, their bodies and movements are immediate evidence of it, but it seems that many of them cannot extend this to form a concept of space in general in which to establish themselves, other people and objects. There is a wealth of literature on this subject, not all of it helpful, but for our purposes the situation can be summed up briefly:

(1) Some children appear to lack the usual ability to understand relationships in three-dimensional space.

(2) In many instances this could be due to lack of free movement

experience in the normal environment.

(3) If, by using a pool, we change this environment in a way which helps movement, they gain in experience.

(4) This should improve their understanding.

Enjoyment

Most children enjoy water, want to learn to swim and have a great sense of achievement as they master the art. They gain in confidence and self-respect and thus benefit socially. In water many handicapped children are better able to compete with normal children and benefit from incentives to improve their stamina and technique. It has been written that 'children suffering from cerebral palsy or muscular dystrophy, amongst other conditions, are blissfully content when they can float; those with a tendency to disregard a malfunctioning limb seem to discover for the first time the body is a complete unit; some children almost change personality when they discard a cumbersome caliper or frame; they blossom . . .' (23) and so the pool plays a part in their overall rehabilitation and total development.

REFERENCE

(23) Duffield, M. H. (Ed) (1969). *Exercises in Water.* London: Ballière, Tindall and Cassell.

Cold therapy

The application of ice, cold packs and other means of reducing temperature is becoming more frequent in some physiotherapy departments as a means of reducing pain, promoting relaxation, improving local circulation and increasing joint range. Many therapists report encouraging results particularly with adults.

The authors, however, have little experience with this treatment in paediatrics except for healing indolent ulcers, when it has proved extremely efficient.

A TREATMENT OUTLINE OF INDIVIDUAL CONDITIONS

A TREATMENT OUTLINE OF INDIVIDUAL CONDITIONS

INTRODUCTION

In Section I our aim has been to give readers a concept of paediatric physiotherapy, so that they may better understand the physiotherapists' role and make best use of what it offers. Each area of treatment was discussed in general terms.

Section II is different. It presents concise details relating to some conditions commonly treated in physiotherapy departments. It cannot be totally inclusive, but we consider that a full range of treatment types has been described. Not all physiotherapists will agree with us, and disagreement is most likely where we consider that:

(1) The advantages of a treatment do not outweigh its disadvantages.

(2) The treatment of a condition is effective, but unnecessary (e.g. muscle strengthening exercises following simple fracture).

(3) Physiotherapy is ineffective.

When we have considered treatment inappropriate, but know of its use in some hospitals, we have noted our doubt.

The disorders are arranged alphabetically and each is dealt with under three headings:

Discussion
References to Section I ⎫ where relevant
Further Reading ⎭

Abscess

Discussion

Those skin abscesses which do not respond to medication may be referred for physiotherapy. The treatment is as for *indolent ulcers.*

Achondroplasia

Discussion

There is usually no indication for physiotherapy. Occasionally young achondroplastic dwarfs with persuasive parents are referred for advice on physical management. If severe bow legs occur and are corrected by osteotomy, post-operative walking training is necessary.

References to Section I

Chapter 2   Chapter 4 (3) (*a*), (*b*)
Chapter 4 (1)   Appendix 1

Further Reading:

Lloyd Roberts, G. C. (1971). *Orthopaedics in Infancy and Childhood.*
    Ed. by J. Apley. London: Butterworths.
Sharrard, W. J. W. (1971). *Paediatric Orthopaedics and Fractures.*
    Oxford and Edinburgh: Blackwell Scientific Publications.

Acne

Discussion

Soap and water, diet and medication are probably the most important factors in treating this distressing condition. Nevertheless some patients respond favourably to irradiation with ultra-violet light. Local exposure to second-degree erythema doses are usually most helpful. Meticulous skin testing for ultra-violet light sensitivity is essential and the physiotherapist must be advised of any contra-indication to irradiation.

References to Section I

Chapter 2
Appendix 7

Further Reading:

Licht, S. (Ed.). (1967). *Therapeutic Electricity and Ultra Violet Radiation.* Elizabeth Licht, New Haven, Conn.

Alopecia

In our experience patients are rarely referred. Irradiation with ultra-violet light is the only treatment physiotherapy can offer.

Alopecia areata

3° erythema doses over small areas sometimes give encouraging results.

Alopecia totalis

A 2° erythema may be beneficial and is a worth-while treatment.

Reference to Section I

Appendix 7

Further Reading:

Licht, S. (Ed.). (1967). *Therapeutic Electricity and Ultra Violet Radiation.* Elizabeth Licht, New Haven, Conn.

Anterior poliomyelitis

Discussion

The authors, in company with many others in this country, have seen no acute cases of APM for several years. They have occasionally seen patients who have a 'polio type' illness and these have been managed physically in the same way as the classical condition. If there is respiratory involvement short- or long-term physiotherapy will be necessary for this particular aspect of the condition.

Acute phase. Nursing positions are most important, splints being used as necessary. Hot wet packs are helpful and gentle passive movements are given daily.

Sub-acute phase. During this period physiotherapy is essential. Assisted active, active and resisted exercises are introduced often using a pool, and the patient's progress recorded by frequent muscle charting. It is impossible to say how long this recovery phase will take. It used to be said that a patient with polio should have treatment until no increase in muscle power was evident and then for a further six months. Since unexpected improvement sometimes occurred during this time, it is a reasonable maxim to follow in this and many neurological conditions.

Orthopaedic phase. There are a number of long-standing cases requiring orthopaedic correction. These need pre-operative functional assessment and post-operative re-education. By this stage of the condition most children have learned trick movements and sometimes manage astonishingly efficient function with very little muscle power. This makes pre-operative assessment particularly difficult and important.

References to Section I

Chapter 2	Chapter 4 (2) (*d*)	Appendix 5
Chapter 3 (Respiration)	Chapter 4 (3) (*a*)	Appendix 6
Chapter 4 (1)	Chapter 4 (3) (*b*)	Appendix 8

Further Reading:

Lloyd Roberts, G. C. (1971). *Orthopaedics in Infancy and Childhood.* Ed. by J. Apley. London: Butterworths.

Bennett, R. L. (1952). 'Physical medicine in poliomyelitis—points of emphasis.' In *Poliomyelitis*, 261–269. Paper at 2nd International Poliomyelitis Conference, Lippincott.

Kettlewell, B. (1956). 'The unique effect of fatigue in poliomyelitis.' *Physiotherapy*, **42**, (2), 45.

Reynolds, R. J. S. (1956). *Physical Measures in the Treatment of Poliomyelitis*. London: Faber and Faber.

Pohl, J. F. and Kenny, E. (1943). *The Kenny Concept of Infantile Paralysis and its Treatment*. St. Paul: Bruce.

Huckstep, R. L. (1970). 'Poliomyelitis in Uganda.' *Physiotherapy*, **56**, (8), 347.

Duffield, M. H. (Ed.) (1969). *Exercises in Water*. London: Baillière, Tindall and Cassell.

Sharrard, W. J. W. (1967). *Paralysis, Upper and Lower Motor Neuron: Clinical Surgery.*, **13**, Orthopaedics London: Butterworths.

Sharrard, W. J. W. (1971). *Paediatric Orthopaedics and Fractures*. Oxford and Edinburgh: Blackwell Scientific Publications.

Arachnodactyly

Discussion

Scoliosis which is a component of this condition is the only indication for physiotherapy. The scoliosis varies from mild to a severity requiring bracing or fusion. The treatment is discussed under scoliosis.

References to Section I

Chapter 2
Chapter 4 (1)

Further Reading:

Lloyd Roberts, G. C. (1971). *Orthopaedics in Infancy and Childhood*. Ed. by J. Apley. London: Butterworths.

Sharrard, W. J. W. (1971). *Paediatric Orthopaedics and Fractures*. Oxford and Edinburgh: Blackwell Scientific Publications.

Arthrogryposis multiplex congenita

Discussion

Physiotherapy should be an early and an important part of the management of this condition, starting as soon as the diagnosis has been made.

The deformities vary and are usually extensive. The children are often intelligent and are therefore able to make full use of any anatomical improvement from surgery.

The aims of physiotherapy are to improve joint range and functional ability. Treatment is by stretching and splinting during the first year of life. After this an assessment of residual deformity can be made and a long-term treatment programme planned. It is necessary for the therapist to consult frequently and regularly with the surgeon. Many years of treatment are inevitable and periodic careful functional assessment, supervision of splinting and calipers, and re-education following surgery should be the responsibility of the therapist. The parents play a large part in the treatment, especially in the first year, and visits to the department should be arranged as frequently as necessary to support the families.

References to Section I

Chapter 2
Chapter 4 (1)
Chapter 4 (3) (*a*)

Chapter 4 (3) (*b*)
Appendix 5

Further Reading:

Lloyd Roberts, G. C. (1971). *Orthopaedics in Infancy and Childhood.* Ed. by J. Apley. London: Butterworths.
Sharrard, W. J. W. (1971). *Paediatric Orthopaedics and Fractures.* Oxford and Edinburgh: Blackwell Scientific Publications.

Asthma

Discussion*

The value of physiotherapy is controversial, some doctors subscribing to it wholeheartedly and others dismissing it vigorously. This means that referrals tend to be haphazard and few comprehensive series have been reported. In a series of 1000 cases the majority of asthmatic children had outgrown the attacks by 16 years, whether

* Over the past few years improved methods of medical treatment with disodium cromoglycate (Intal) and beclomethasone dipropionate aerosol have become available and are likely to improve the prognosis

they had physiotherapy or not. However, the follow up of 5 to 16 years showed a significant difference favouring those who had received physiotherapy; they were subsequently less prone to bronchitis and postural problems (Kiernander, 1972). As there is no way at the moment of telling which children will benefit, it is not unreasonable to suggest that physiotherapy should be tried in all cases that are not making an immediately satisfactory response to medication. Effective physiotherapy may help the doctor to keep medical treatments to a minimum (Apley and Mac Keith, 1968).

The aims of treatment are: (*a*) to maintain chest mobility; (*b*) to improve the breathing pattern, by diminishing attempted forceful expiration; (*c*) to promote relaxation, including teaching positions useful during an attack; (*d*) to improve posture; (*e*) to increase exercise tolerance.

It follows that the appropriate time for physiotherapy is between attacks and a long training programme may be required. The rationale of treatment must be carefully explained to the family. A child having an asthma attack is frightened and unless he has previously been well trained will often require antispasmodic therapy.

The therapist needs to know of any discovered allergies and of social conditions which may influence the problem. A suitable programme can then be instituted.

Asthmatic children are among the most difficult referred for physiotherapy. They require therapists who are experienced, patient, but above all honest enough to recognize when the children are not responding.

REFERENCES

Apley, J. and Mac Keith, R. (1968). *The Child and His Symptoms*, p.45. Oxford and Edinburgh. Blackwell Scientific Publications.
Kiernander, B. (1972). Personal communication.

References to Section I

Chapter 2   Appendix 8
Chapter 3

Further Reading:

Groen, J. J. (1972). 'The mechanism of the disturbance of respiration during the asthmatic attack.' *Physiotherapy*, **58**, (11), 371.
Kiernander, B. (Ed.) (1965). *Physical Medicine in Paediatrics*. London: Butterworths.

Bacterial infections

Discussion

The vast majority of bacterial infections do not require physiotherapy. There are those however when chest complications may present as primary or secondary symptoms, e.g. brucellosis, pertussis. If physiotherapy is indicated in these situations it should proceed as described for medical chest conditions.

If the bacterial infection involves the nervous system it should be treated by physiotherapy symptomatically at the appropriate time.

Reference to Section I

Chapter 3 (4)

Benign congenital hypotonia

Discussion

This is an outdated term now generally abandoned. It included a number of conditions and some of the children so labelled turned out later to have serious lasting disorders. Many children had nothing more than a degree of hypotonia, bottom shuffling rather tnan crawling, delay in walking, and later flat feet and knock knees. As any of these may cause parental concern it is helpful to give advice on handling. In a minority still mistakenly referred with this diagnosis severe deformity occurs and these children will often require orthopaedic intervention and therefore pre-operative functional assessment and post-operative training.

References to Section I

Chapter 2	Chapter 4 (3) (*a*)	Appendix 5
Chapter 4 (1)	Chapter 4 (3) (*b*)	Appendix 6
	Appendix 1	Appendix 8

Further Reading:

Dubowitz, V. (1968). 'The myopathies.' *Physiotherapy*, **54**, (11), 384.
Walton, J. N. (1956). 'Benign congenital hypotonia.' *Lancet* **1**, 1023.

Blindness

Discussion

Massive sensory deprivation in infancy has widespread effects on motor development and other sensory experience. From the earliest age management of their physical environment will influence the children's achievements. To this aspect of their management the paediatric physiotherapy department can make a major contribution and should be consulted at the earliest stage. These children can usually be included in a special nursery group and the parents and staff taught how to handle them appropriately.

See Deafness

References to Section I

| Chapter 2 | Appendix 3 | Appendix 6 |
| Appendix 1 | Appendix 4 | Appendix 8 |

Boils and carbuncles

Discussion

It is almost unknown for boils and carbuncles to be treated in a children's department. If exceptionally the area becomes indolent treatment may proceed as for an indolent ulcer.

Although still referred to in some text-books, general or local irradiation with ultra-violet light has been largely superseded by other therapies.

Bronchiectasis

Discussion

Patients do sometimes present with bronchiectasis although much less often than in the past. The main aims of treatment are to clear the lungs of secretions and treatment should proceed as for cystic fibrosis with frank lung involvement.

See Cystic fibrosis

Burns

Discussion

Treatment of burns varies from unit to unit. The physiotherapist's role is seen as essential, incidental or irrelevant. We think that physiotherapists have a valuable contribution to make and that in any unit in which their help is ever needed they should work as part of a team rather than an 'extra' for special occasions.

Important aims of treatment are to prevent chest complications, hasten healing and restore function. In the acute stage chest care, positioning and possibly splinting are the therapist's main concern. Gentle assisted-active and active movements, massage to stable strip grafts, general mobilizing and pool therapy are introduced as appropriate.

References to Section I

Chapter 3 (Respiratory)   Appendix 8
Appendix 5

Further Reading:

Trussell, E. C. and Hayne, J. C. R. (1970). 'Physiotherapy in the treatment of burns and plastic surgery.' *Physiotherapy*, **56**, (3), 150.
Duffield, M. H. (Ed.) (1969). *Exercises in Water*. London: Baillière, Tindall and Cassell.

Cerebral accidents

Discussion

The physiotherapist has two distinct roles in relation to (1) respiratory and (2) movement and general stimulation. She will need to know the date of the incident, the areas of lung collapse and of any disorder other than those of cerebral origin.

Respiratory

The aim of treatment is to improve ventilation and the means are 'passive' breathing exercises combined with percussion/vibrations.

References to Section I

Chapter 2
Chapter 3

Movement and general stimulation

Treatment should be started while the patient is unconscious. It is essential to prevent contractures if movement ability is not to be restricted later. As movement recovery begins the child needs progressively greater postural and movement demands made upon him.
See also Road traffic accidents

References to Section I

Chapter 2	Appendix 1	Appendix 5
Chapter 4 (1)	Appendix 2	Appendix 6
Chapter 4 (2) (*a*)	Appendix 3	

Further Reading:

Brink, J. D., Garrett, A. L., Hale, W. R., Woo-Sam, J. and Nickel, V. L. (1970). 'Recovery of motor and intellectual function in children sustaining severe head injuries.' *Dev. Med. Child. Neurol.*, **12**, 565.
See also Cerebral Palsy—Further Reading

Cerebral Palsy

Discussion

The treatment of this condition varies with the type of movement disorder, age, intelligence, previous treatment and many other (including domestic) factors. The physiotherapist needs to be advised of the probable cause and of any other disorders (particularly mental retardation, hearing, visual and epilepsy). Since the treatment depends upon the presenting signs, no more precise diagnosis than 'cerebral palsy' is mandatory. The more the physiotherapist is kept in the picture the more she can help; both directly and indirectly through the parents.

References to Section I

Further Reading:

Blockley, J. and Miller, G. (1971). 'Feeding techniques with cerebral-palsied children.' *Physiotherapy*, **57**, (7), 300.

'An Exploratory and Analytical Survey of Therapeutic Exercise.' (1966). North West Univ: Special Therapeutic Exercise Project. *Am. J. Phys. Med.*, **46**, (1), 1967.

Bobath, K. and Bobath, B. (1964). 'The facilitation of normal postural reactions and movements in the treatment of cerebral palsy.' *Physiotherapy*, **50**, (8), 246.

Bobath, B. (1967). 'The very early treatment of cerebral palsy.' *Dev. Med. Child. Neurol.*, **9**, (4), 373.

Brunnstrom, S. (1956). *Methods Used to Elicit, Reinforce and Co-ordinate Muscular Response in Upper Motor Neuron Lesions. Am. Phys. Ther. Ass.*, O.V.R., Institute Papers. New York: American Physical Therapy Association.

Cotton, E. (1970). 'Integration of treatment and education in cerebral palsy.' *Physiotherapy*, **56**, (4), 143.

Cotton, E. (1965). 'The Institute of Movement Therapy and School for "Conductors" Budapest, Hungary.' *Dev. Med. Child. Neurol.*, **7**, 437.

Halpern, D., Kottke, F. J., Burrill, C., Fiterman, C., Popp, J. and Palmer, S. (1970). 'Training of control of head posture in children with cerebral palsy.' *Dev. Med. Child. Neurol.*, **12**, 290.

Knott, M. and Voss, D. E. (1968). *Proprioceptive neuro-muscular facilitation.* New York: Harper Row.

Rood, M. (1967). 'Miss Rood's approach.' *Am. J. phys. Med.*, **46**, 1.

Goff, B. (1969). 'Appropriate afferent stimulation.' *Physiotherapy*, **55**, (1), 9.

Holt, K. S. (1965). *Assessment of Cerebral Palsy.* 1. London: Lloyd-Luke (Medical Books).

Holt, K. S. and Reynell, J. K. (1967). *Assessment of Cerebral Palsy.* 2. London: Lloyd-Luke (Medical Books).

Christmas disease

See Haemophilia and Christmas disease

Chronic degenerative neurological conditions

Discussion

Some children are referred for management even although it is recognized from the outset that their condition—possibly without any specific diagnosis—is degenerative. It is often possible to make their lives more tolerable by teaching the parents how to handle them and perhaps by providing aids and appliances. Parents require continuing practical support and we consider this to be a proper function of a paediatric physiotherapist.

References to Section I

Chapter 2   Chapter 4 (1)   Appendix 6
Chapter 3 (Respiration)   Chapter 4 (2) (*a*)

Congenital dislocation of the hip

Discussion

Congenital dislocation of the hip treated conservatively very seldom requires physiotherapy. It may be the physiotherapist's role to advise on a suitable chair or trolley for use if the child is in a frog plaster or abduction splint. There are several excellent devices available but in most cases a small chair or stool with its legs cut down and fitted with castors so that the child's feet can reach the floor is eminently suitable. Very occasionally the child's legs do not 'come down' from the position of immobilization and then a short period of suitable exercises and parental instruction may be needed. Mobilization exercises are necessary following surgery. In the majority of cases the course of treatment will be short; in a few, hip and knee stiffness persist, necessitating prolonged intensive physiotherapy.

References to Section I

Chapter 4 (1)
Chapter 4 (3) (*b*)

Further Reading:

Lloyd Roberts, G. C. (1971). *Orthopaedics in Infancy and Childhood.*
    Ed. by J. Apley. London: Butterworths.
Sharrard, W. J. W. (1971). *Paediatric Orthopaedics and Fractures.*
    Oxford and Edinburgh: Blackwell Scientific Publications.

Congenital elevation of the fifth toe

Discussion

Stretching and corrective strapping is helpful.

References to Section I

Chapter 2	Chapter 4 (3) (*c*)
Chapter 4 (1)	Appendix 5

Further Reading:

Lloyd Roberts, G. C. (1971). *Orthopaedics in Infancy and Childhood.*
    Ed. by J. Apley. London: Butterworths.
Sharrard, W. J. W. (1971). *Paediatric Orthopaedics and Fractures.*
    Oxford and Edinburgh: Blackwell Scientific Publications.

Congenital heart disorder

Discussion

The physiotherapist's main role here is in respiratory care following surgery. Hemiplegia may be a complication of congenital heart
disorder and occasionally occurs post-operatively. The treatment
will be as for acute hemiplegia, suitably modified during immediate
post-operative period.

Reference to Section I

Chapter 3

Congenital malformations: larynx, trachea and oesophagus

Discussion

When these conditions are treated surgically they will require intensive post-operative chest physiotherapy, unless there are over-riding contraindications.

Reference to Section I

Chapter 3

Congenital malformations—parental concern

Discussion

There is a variety of congenital deformities, e.g. Pectus excavatus and Klippel–Feil deformity which although not themselves amenable to any form of physiotherapy, nevertheless will benefit from general stimulation if gross movements are in any way affected. The parents are understandably worried by any of these conditions. A few visits to a therapist and contact with a physiotherapy department to be instructed in general handling and management are to the family's, and therefore the child's advantage.

Reference to Section I

Chapter 2

Conversion hysteria

Discussion

Accurate diagnosis will eliminate children with habit spasm or tic. (In general a tic is best ignored while the problems of the child and his family are looked into by the paediatrician. The less notice taken of a tic the more quickly it will go away.) Nevertheless, conversion hysteria is a real disorder and in a small number of cases the physiotherapist has a useful part to play in management after referral from a psychiatrist. It is essential that these children are treated in or at a specialist psychiatric unit which has ready access to a paediatric physiotherapy department.

Reference to Section I

Chapter 4 (1)

Curly toes

Discussion

These often correct with growth. Strapping is not thought to influence the eventual outcome but may be useful initially so that shoes can be worn without discomfort.

References to Section I

Chapter 2	Chapter 4 (3) (*c*)
Chapter 4 (1)	Appendix 5 (p. 116)

Further Reading:

Lloyd Roberts, G. C. (1971). *Orthopaedics in Infancy and Childhood.* Ed. by J. Apley. London: Butterworths.
Sharrard, W. J. W. (1971). *Paediatric Orthopaedics and Fractures.* Oxford and Edinburgh: Blackwell Scientific Publications.

Cystic fibrosis

Discussion

Early diagnosis and improved medical treatment have dramatically altered the prognosis of this inherited disease. Lung involvement is still the major problem and the most usual cause of death. All children with cystic fibrosis should be referred for physiotherapy immediately on diagnosis, even if there are no clinical signs of lung involvement (Norman, 1973). The aim here is to help to keep the lung tissue healthy and general exercise will be emphasized. Postural drainage assisted by percussion is usually an obvious need as the most efficient way to remove the tenacious mucus produced in this condition. Specific breathing exercises may be necessary if there are areas of collapse. Expert and prolonged medical care and parental support are of paramount importance.

The therapist must have the most recent x-ray report available so that she can select the appropriate drainage positions and breathing exercises. She must also know the current medical treatment; for instance, if inhalations are included, physiotherapy will be arranged at the most efficient times.

Some children with cystic fibrosis have nasal polyps which are very troublesome, causing blocked sinuses and adding to the danger of intercurrent infection. A course of short-wave diathermy following surgical removal of polyps has recently been introduced routinely. To date we have not treated many cases but the results so far are promising. The polyps have not recurred and sinus drainage has improved.

REFERENCE

Norman, A. P. (1973). Personal communication.

References to Section I

Chapter 2   Appendix 8
Chapter 3

Further Reading:

Young, W. F. (1967). 'Cystic fibrosis.' *Physiotherapy*, **53** (2), 48.
Burton, L. (1972). 'An investigation into the problems occasioned for the child with cystic fibrosis.' In *Proceedings of 84th Annual General Meeting of I.C.A.A.*
Rubin, S. (1967). 'Physiotherapy and cystic fibrosis.' *Physiotherapy*, **53**, (2), 51.
Morony, T. (1969). 'Cystic fibrosis.' *Austr. J. Phys.*, **XV**, (4), 125.

Deafness

Discussion

Although in some respects as great a handicap as blindness, deafness has little effect on movement development. However, these children not infrequently come under the wing of a physiotherapist because the parents need advice about play or because the child is in a special care unit which already has physiotherapy supervision. In theory this role is more suited to the speech therapist, but they are few and far between.

When a deaf child has some other handicap (for example, cerebral palsy) there can be great problems in treatment, particularly post-operatively. In spite of every effort to tell him about it, the operation may have taken him by surprise. The physiotherapist may have difficulty in explaining what she requires of the child and it is hard to give reassurance that he is not to be 'assaulted' yet again.

See Blindness.

Dermatomysositis

See Myositis

Encephalitis

See Cerebral accidents

Facial nerve palsy

Discussion

Few patients benefit from referral to a physiotherapy department. Some children, who can tolerate adequate electrical stimulation benefit noticeably from this treatment. It is useful and reassuring to teach a simple scheme of facial exercises which can be practised as a game at home.

See Peripheral nerve injuries

Flat foot

Discussion

Mobile painless non-paralytic flat feet do not require physiotherapy. They often cause family concern and if so a simple test, to reassure the parents that all muscles are working normally, is all that is required. If a child can walk on his heels, toes, inner and outer borders of his feet he clearly has balanced muscle group action, and if a full range of passive movements can also be demonstrated there is no cause for concern. Over the years teaching unnecessary 'remedial' exercises to normal feet has wasted time in many physiotherapy departments.

Slack posture, when children stand with hips internally rotated, may cause feet to fall into valgus and can be counteracted by a scheme of general exercises. Co-operation with schools and school medical services should help to keep such children away from hospital.

Painful flat feet. If the pain is severe enough to necessitate rest, non-weight-bearing exercises may be helpful.

Paralytic flat feet may present as a result of poliomyelitis, spinal lesions or cerebral palsy and should be treated as part of the whole condition.

References to Section I

Chapter 2   Appendix 5 (p. 116)
Chapter 4 (1)

Further Reading:

Lloyd Roberts, G. C. (1971). *Orthopaedics in Infancy and Childhood.* Ed. by J. Apley. London: Butterworths.

Gray, E. R. (1969). 'The role of leg muscles in variations of the arches in normal and flat feet.' *Phys. Ther.,* **49**, 10, 1084.

Bleck, E. E. (1971). 'The shoeing of children: sham or science?' *Dev. Med. Child. Neurol.,* **13**, 188.

Sharrard, W. J. W. (1971). *Paediatric Orthopaedics and Fractures.* Oxford and Edinburgh: Blackwell Scientific Publications.

Foot deformities

See Congenital elevation of the fifth toe; Curly toes; Flat foot; Hallux valgus; Metatarsus varus; Pes cavus; Talipes

Fractures

Discussion

The vast majority of fractures sustained in childhood require no physiotherapy. If there is any nerve involvement this will be treated as in '*peripheral nerve injuries*'.

References to Section I

Chapter 4 (1)
Chapter 4 (3) (*d*)

Further Reading:

Sharrard, W. J. W. (1971). *Paediatric Orthopaedics and Fractures.*
   p. 930. Oxford and Edinburgh: Blackwell Scientific Publications.

Genu valgum

Discussion

Idiopathic Knock Knee.—The parents need reassuring that the
condition requires neither exercises nor splinting. The orthopaedic
surgeon will have taught the parents to measure the distance between
the malleoli when the child is lying on his back with knees together.
The condition will only require further investigation if the interval
increases as the child grows.

Secondary Knock Knee (e.g. spina bifida, endocrine disturbances,
rheumatoid arthritis).—This will almost certainly require splinting,
exercises and possibly post-operative re-education. It should be
considered as part of the general condition and not in isolation.

References to Section I

Chapter 2
Chapter 4 (1)

Further Reading:

Lloyd Roberts, G. C. (1971). *Orthopaedics in Infancy and Childhood.*
   Ed. by J. Apley. London: Butterworths.
Sharrard, W. J. W. (1971). *Paediatric Orthopaedics and Fractures.*
   Oxford and Edinburgh: Blackwell Scientific Publications.

Haemophilia and Christmas disease

Discussion

Patients with these conditions are seen less frequently in physiotherapy departments since recent advances in haematological control. Prolonged periods as an inpatient and immobilization are no

longer necessary. The principles of physiotherapy are however precisely the same as before. Rest in the acute phase following a bleed (usually only two days); then, starting with pool therapy, a carefully graded scheme of exercises is designed to increase muscle strength and restore the range of movement. The knee joint is the most troublesome. It is important that exercises are continued at home. Resting splints and prolonged plastering are now rarely used.

It should be emphasized however that treatment must be started immediately a bleed occurs. Severe contractures may develop within a few days in a neglected joint and then manipulation and plastering or even open surgery may be necessary.

References to Section I

Chapter 4 (1)   Chapter 4 (3) (b)   Appendix 8
Chapter 4 (3) (a)   Appendix 5

Further Reading:

Greg, G. (1964). 'The haemophiliac joint and its treatment by physical methods.' *Physiotherapy*, **50**, (12), 394.
Duffield, M. H. (Ed.) (1969). *Exercises in Water*. London: Baillière, Tindall and Cassell.
Sharrard, W. J. W. (1971). *Paediatric Orthopaedics and Fractures.* Oxford and Edinburgh: Blackwell Scientific Publications.

Hallux valgus

Discussion

Although hallux valgus unaccompanied by any other disorder may be mild and symptom free in childhood it should be watched carefully for deterioration or pain. Surgery may then be indicated and prevent considerable trouble in adult life. Foot exercises are unlikely to be of specific benefit, but, post-operatively, exercises and walking training are essential.

In cerebral palsy or myelomeningocoele, however, hallux valgus frequently causes trophic ulceration or pain. Indeed this is often the only vigorous complaint of an ambulant patient with cerebral palsy. The solution is to be found in surgery at the appropriate age followed by meticulous post-operative physiotherapy.

In a very few instances strapping into abduction may help to relieve symptoms but surgery will still be needed; the object primarily being to make it more comfortable to wear shoes so that the effect of the deformity on the walking pattern is minimized.

References to Section I

Chapter 2   Chapter 4 (3) (*a*) (*b*)
Chapter 4 (1)

Further Reading:

Lloyd Roberts, G. C. (1971). *Orthopaedics in Infancy and Childhood.*
    Ed. by J. Apley. London: Butterworths.
Sharrard, W. J. W. (1971). *Paediatric Orthopaedics and Fractures.*
    Oxford and Edinburgh: Blackwell Scientific Publications.

Hurler syndrome—gargoylism (and similar syndromes)

Discussion

There is a considerable variation in the severity of this syndrome. The children usually have delayed locomotor milestones and their unresponsiveness is the despair of their parents, who require support and encouragement. We have found that an experienced physiotherapist is often the best person to provide the necessary practical help for the child and support for the family. The physiotherapist can do much for the child with delay in motor development.

References to Section I

Chapter 2   Appendix 1   Appendix 5
Chapter 4 (1)   Appendix 2   Appendix 6
Chapter 4 (2) (*a*)   Appendix 3   Appendix 8
Chapter 4 (2) (*b*)   Appendix 4

Further Reading:

Lloyd Roberts, G. C. (1971). *Orthopaedics in Infancy and Childhood.*
    Ed. by J. Apley. London: Butterworths.
Sharrard, W. J. W. (1971). *Paediatric Orthopaedics and Fractures.*
    Oxford and Edinburgh: Blackwell Scientific Publications.

Indolent ulcers

Discussion

Indolent ulcers occur most commonly where there is deficient sensation and are therefore seen usually in children with spina bifida.

A crumpled sock, ill-fitting shoe or caliper may cause friction and the skin will break down easily and the area quickly becomes indolent. The aim of treatment is to improve the circulation as speedily and vigorously as possible in order to promote healing. Apart from her own observation of the area, the only information the therapist requires is to know if the child is a self-mutilator as this may influence treatment. Large doses of ultra-violet light to the open area and 2nd degree erythema to the surrounding skin will often speed healing. Alternatively the application of crushed ice has proved effective and has the advantage of being a treatment easily carried out at home.

References to Section I

Chapter 2   Appendix 7
Appendix 5

Further Reading:

Licht, S. (1965). 'Local cryotherapy.' In *Therapeutic Heat and Cold.* Ed. by S. Licht, Elizabeth Licht, New Haven, Conn.
Marshall, R. S. (1971). 'Cold therapy in the treatment of pressure sores.' *Physiotherapy*, **57**, (8), 372.
Licht, S. (Ed.) (1967). *Therapeutic Electricity and Ultra Violet Radiation.* Elizabeth Licht, New Haven, Conn.

Larynx

See Congenital malformations

Meningitis

Discussion

Meningitis in the newborn and during the first year is not uncommonly followed by cerebral palsy, mental handicap or epilepsy.

After the age of one, if treated early, the outlook is good. The permanent results of meningitis are sometimes more grave than those of encephalitis. The aims and means of physiotherapy for both these conditions are similar.

See Cerebral accidents   ·

Mental deficiency

Discussion

Mental deficiency is a frequent cause of motor developmental delay and physiotherapy should be started in infancy. Many children with mild retardation and all with severe mental deficiency benefit from physiotherapy. Many non-ambulant children continue to benefit from treatment until the apparent limit of their motor ability is reached, after which supervision of posture may be of continued importance. The physiotherapist needs to know the probable cause, age of onset and any other disorder (particularly movement, vision, hearing, epilepsy).

References to Section I

Chapter 2	Appendix 1	Appendix 4
Chapter 4 (1)	Appendix 2	Appendix 5
Chapter 4 (2) (*b*)	Appendix 3	Appendix 6

Further Reading:

Campbell, E. D. R. and Green, E. A. (1970). 'Treatment of cerebral palsy in the severely subnormal.' *Rheum. Phys. Med.* **X**, 8.
Hughes, N. A. S. (1971). 'Developmental physiotherapy for mentally handicapped babies.' *Physiotherapy,* **57**, (9), 399.
Illingworth, R. S. (1966). *The Development of the Infant and Young Child, Normal and Abnormal.* Edinburgh and London: Livingstone.
Milani-Comparetti, A. and Gidoni, E. A. (1967). 'Routine developmental examination in normal and retarded children.' *Dev. Med. Child. Neurol.,* **9**, 631.

Metatarsus varus

Discussion

There are various degrees of deformity. Physiotherapy is unnecessary for the mildest, which are self-correcting by muscle action alone. With greater deformity the aim is to restore the foot to normal alignment and this can usually be achieved by teaching the parents how to stretch the forefoot into valgus. For the few requiring surgery a short period of post-operative re-education is required.

References to Section I

Chapter 4 (3) (*a*)   Appendix 5 (p. 116)
Chapter 4 (3) (*b*)

Further Reading:

Lloyd Roberts, G. C. (1971). *Orthopaedics in Infancy and Childhood.* Ed. by J. Apley. London: Butterworths.
Sharrard, W. J. W. (1971). *Paediatric Orthopaedics and Fractures.* Oxford and Edinburgh: Blackwell Scientific Publications.

Mouth breathers

Discussion

Some small children keep their mouths open while breathing through the nose, but some children are habitual mouth breathers. Mouth breathing—failure to maintain an 'oral seal' during breathing —has a variety of causes and all children referred to a physiotherapist (or speech therapist) should have been examined by an E.N.T. surgeon and, possibly, a dentist. It is doubtful that there is a simple relationship between total body posture and oral posture, but a relationship of sorts exists: mouth breathers frequently have slack and drooping general posture. Most physiotherapists teach the young child to blow his nose (many children of five cannot do this adequately) and then encourage him to join in games and exercises to promote normal posture and better ventilation. Exercise, which *encourages* mouth breathing, may appear out of place but physiotherapists treat the child's posture and approach to life as a whole *to prevent habitual bad posture* rather than the specific referred 'disability'. It is helpful if there is contact with the school so that super-vision can be continued without interfering with ordinary life.

References to Section I

Chapter 2
Chapter 3

Muscular dystrophy

Discussion

Whilst physiotherapy is powerless to prevent the inevitable pro-gression of this group of disorders it has a large part to play in the general physical management of the whole family. The therapist needs to know the type of muscular dystrophy, the prognosis, precise-ly what the parents have been told of the condition and its likely outcome, and of any other disorder.

Treatment is concerned with two distinct functions: movement, which is likely to take precedence when the child is young; and respiration, which is of greater importance in the later stages.

Movement. Exercise programmes must be carefully designed to avoid fatigue and sitting posture should be watched carefully. It is particularly important that, when a wheelchair becomes necessary, the most suitable available is provided. The aims of treatment are to limit deformity and to maintain mobility and general activity, so helping the child to make the most of his diminishing abilities.

References to Section I

Chapter 2   Chapter 4 (2) (*d*)   Appendix 6
Chapter 4 (1)   Appendix 5   Appendix 8

Further Reading:

Dubowitz, V. (1968). 'The myopathies.' *Physiotherapy*, **54**, (11), 384.
Walton, J. N. (1956). 'Benign congenital hypotonia.' *Lancet* **1**, 1023.
Sharrard, W. J. W. (1971). *Paediatric Orthopaedics and Fractures.* Oxford and Edinburgh: Blackwell Scientific Publications.

Respiration Respiration difficulties are common in the later stages of this disease. The physiotherapist needs to know the diagnosis and the areas of lung collapse. The aim of treatment will be to keep the airways clear, and incidentally, help relieve the intense fear of suffocation experienced by many of these children. This requires postural drainage, percussion and both active and passive exercises.

Reference to Section I

Chapter 3

Myositis

Discussion

The aims and means of physical treatment in this condition can be considered together. The treatment is best considered in relation to two phases.

Acute phase. There is extreme muscular tenderness. Fixed deformity occurs readily and it is therefore essential to nurse the patient in a carefully supervised resting position, and also to move all joints daily through as full a range as pain allows. Bed cradles and splints are helpful; lightweight plastic materials are preferred for splintage as they cause less pain during moulding and application.

Sub-acute phase. The aim is to encourage mobility; assisted-active and active movements combined with pool therapy, together form the most pleasant and efficient method; heated paraffin wax can also be used (Millard, 1965). The therapist needs to know the time of onset of the illness *and* to be advised of the medical management of the patient.

REFERENCE

Millard, J. B. (1965). 'Conductive heating' in *Therapeutic Heat and Cold*. Ed. S. Licht, Eliz. Licht Newhaven, Conn.

References to Section I

Chapter 4 (1)   Appendix 5
Chapter 4 (2) (*d*)   Appendix 8

Further Reading:

Kiernander, B. (Ed.) (1965). *Physical Medicine in Paediatrics*. London: Butterworths.

Myositis ossificans traumatica

Discussion

Now rarely seen, it most usually affects the elbow joint and must be treated with great respect. Carefully graduated exercise can sometimes be helpful.

References to Section I

Chapter 4 (1)
Chapter 4 (3) (*e*)

Further Reading:

Lloyd Roberts, G. C. (1971). *Orthopaedics in Infancy and Childhood.* Ed. by J. Apley. London: Butterworths.

Neurological conditions, chronic degenerative

See Chronic degenerative neurological conditions

Obstetrical paralysis of the brachial plexus (Erb, Klumpke and Mixed)

Discussion

It is not always easy to determine the precise degree of paralysis in the neonate, since the arm usually lies immobile. As the baby gets older an accurate muscle chart should be attempted as an aid to planning further management. The aim of physiotherapy is similar in all cases: to prevent fixed deformity.

It is *not necessary* to splint the arm into abduction, but a wrist cock-up splint may very occasionally be helpful. The mother is taught appropriate passive movements and stretchings, particular attention being paid to external rotation of the shoulder. These should be performed at least twice a day. As much active movement as possible should be encouraged. As soon as the family is confident about doing the movements frequent visits to a physiotherapy department are unnecessary; monthly checks are usually adequate.

Unresolved cases which require surgery will need post-operative movement education.

References to Section I

Chapter 2   Chapter 4 (2) (*d*)
Chapter 4 (1)

Further Reading:

Lloyd Roberts, G. C. (1971). *Orthopaedics in Infancy and Childhood.*
    Ed. by J. Apley. London: Butterworths.

Oesophagus

See Congenital malformations

Osteogenesis imperfecta

Discussion

    The need for physiotherapy varies with the severity of the condi-
tion. Some children escape with few fractures and rarely find their
way to physiotherapy departments; others spend a large proportion
of their lives in hospital. Physiotherapy is directed towards improving function and guarding against fracture. Protective splinting,
often using proprietary thermo-plastic materials, may be necessary.
Pool therapy is one of the most useful methods of mobilization. The
patient is almost always apprehensive of movement and it is therefore most desirable that the same therapist should continue to treat
him.

References to Section I

Chapter 2   Chapter 4 (3) (*a*)   Appendix 5
Chapter 4 (1)   Chapter 4 (3) (*b*)   Appendix 8

Further Reading:

Lloyd Roberts, G. C. (1971). *Orthopaedics in Infancy and Childhood.*
    Ed. by J. Apley. London: Butterworths.
Duffield, M. H. (Ed.) (1969). *Exercises in Water.* London: Baillière,
    Tindall and Cassell.
Sharrard, W. J. W. (1971). *Paediatric Orthopaedics and Fractures.*
    Oxford and Edinburgh: Blackwell Scientific Publications.

Peripheral nerve injuries

Discussion

Any peripheral nerve may be involved. Some of the commonest are sited in the forearm following such injuries as pushing a hand through a window.

Referral for physiotherapy is always necessary for suitable splinting and functional re-education. In addition to passive movements and active exercises a few *older* patients benefit from electrical stimulation.

Intensive treatment is required particularly following suture; admission to hospital solely for physiotherapy being occasionally justified. Parental co-operation is most important as these children tend to be incident prone.

References to Section I

Chapter 2   Chapter 4 (2) (*d*)   Chapter 4 (3) (*b*)
Chapter 4 (1)   Chapter 4 (3) (*a*)   Appendix 5

Pes cavus

Discussion

Idiopathic Pes Cavus.   Physiotherapy is unnecessary.
Secondary Pes Cavus (e.g. spina bifida occulta). The therapist may be asked for a functional assessment, and will be involved in rehabilitation after surgery.

References to Section I

Chapter 4 (1)   Chapter 4 (3) (*b*)
Chapter 4 (3) (*a*)

Further Reading:

Lloyd Roberts, G. C. (1971). *Orthopaedics in Infancy and Childhood.*
   Ed. by J. Apley. London: Butterworths.
Sharrard, W. J. W. (1971). *Paediatric Orthopaedics and Fractures.*
   Oxford and Edinburgh: Blackwell Scientific Publications.

Phocomelia

Discussion

Management should be directed towards establishing the greatest independence for the patient. In spite of this there is a general tendency for children to be assessed at as early an age as possible for the fitting of prostheses even if these are less efficient than the existing rudimentary limb. The authors think that with upper limb involvement children are often better off and happier uncluttered by prostheses. This may also be true for some of those with lower limb involvement.

A single lower limb prosthesis is usually accepted willingly and children require very little training, except in skin care and application of the limb.

In view of the general public's inability to accept disfigured people in the community the patient and family need continuous support.

References to Section I

Chapter 2	Appendix 1	Appendix 5
Chapter 4 (1)	Appendix 3	

Further Reading:

Lloyd Roberts, G. C. (1971). *Orthopaedics in Infancy and Childhood.* Ed. by J. Apley. London: Butterworths.

Catto, A. M. and MacNaughton, A. (1966). 'Physiotherapy and occupational therapy in the management of the upper limb amputee.' *Physiotherapy*, **52**, (6), 187.

Pearson, F. A. and Spiers, B. W. (1966). 'Teamwork in the management of dysmelic children.' *Physiotherapy*, **52**, (6), 197.

Brooks, M. B. (1969). 'Success and failure in infant prosthetic fitting.' *Rehabilitation*, **70**, 31.

Kiernander, B. (Ed.) (1965). *Physical Medicine in Paediatrics.* London: Butterworths.

Sharrard, W. J. W. (1971). *Paediatric Orthopaedics and Fractures.* Oxford and Edinburgh: Blackwell Scientific Publications.

Poliomyelitis, anterior

See Anterior poliomyelitis

Polyneuritis

Discussion

In children polyneuritis is usually an illness of acute onset; relapses often occur during the course of the illness. Most make a complete recovery. Physiotherapy is an important part of management throughout.

Acute phase. Respiratory care is vital. Patients may be on a respirator and physiotherapy is needed, and may be necessary as frequently as two hourly.

Splinting, particularly of the feet, and careful passive movements must be started immediately to prevent deformity occurring. A muscle chart should be completed early as a base-line for future assessment.

Recovery phase. Graded exercises and re-education of active movement will start as soon as the general condition of the patient allows and pool therapy is helpful. Periodic muscle charting will help to determine when the condition is quiescent.

Consistent and intensive physical management during the full course of the disease should eliminate the need for surgery to correct deformity.

Surgery is occasionally necessary, but is not undertaken until the condition appears completely static.

Post-operative physiotherapy will proceed as appropriate.

References to Section I

Chapter 2	Chapter 4 (2) (*d*)	Appendix 6
Chapter 3 (Respiratory)	Appendix 5	Appendix 8
Chapter 4 (1)		

Further Reading:

Duffield, M. H. (Ed.) (1969). *Exercises in Water*. London: Baillière, Tindall and Cassell.
Kiernander, B. (Ed.) (1965). *Physical Medicine in Paediatrics*. London: Butterworths.

Posture

Discussion

There is no one perfect posture to suit everybody, therefore it might be argued that general postural exercises have little value. However, a good posture is an efficient posture, efficient in differing circumstances, implying adaptability, and so mobility. This is not to say that all children should attend physiotherapy departments or remedial classes for general postural exercises, which could well be— but are not usually—part of the school curriculum. Nevertheless, gross disturbances of posture do intrude into many conditions; for instance the fixed, round shouldered, rigid posture of a child with a chronic chest condition, or the raised shoulder of a baby with a sterno-mastoid tumour.

Each child with locomotor difficulty requiring physiotherapy should be looked at as a complete person and mobilizing postural exercises included in the treatment programme.

References to Section I

Chapter 2
Chapter 4 (1)

Further Reading:

Kiernander, B. (Ed.) (1965). *Physical Medicine in Paediatrics.* London: Butterworths.
Asher, D. (1974). *Postural Variations in Childhood.* London: Butterworths.

Pressure sores

Discussion

Despite great care pressure sores do sometimes occur in children. They should be treated as indolent ulcers.
See Indolent ulcers

Psoriasis

Discussion

There is a considerable variation in the type and distribution of lesion in this condition, and these vary from small pinkish patches to large red scaly areas which often crack and become sore. The lesions occur on any area of the body, although they are uncommon on the face.

Treatment has varied over the years; tar preparations being considered extremely effective at some times and positively dangerous at others. It is our experience that, according to the type of lesion, exposure to sub-erythema, 1°E or 2°E doses of UVL combined with tar baths or other tar preparations are often helpful. We have never found high-frequency current treatment, which is recommended in some literature, helpful in treating scalp lesions.

In general, psoriasis can be dealt with on an outpatient basis but short periods in hospital for intensive treatment may be justified.

Usually both the children and their parents are extremely worried by this condition and need to be reassured that it is not contagious or infectious, and that hair will not fall out. In children of school age it is essential that teachers understand the nature of the condition as children sometimes suffer considerable rejection and teasing by their peers.

References to Section I

Chapter 2
Appendix 7

Further Reading:

Licht, S. (Ed.) (1967). *Therapeutic Electricity and Ultra Violet Radiation.* Elizabeth Licht, New Haven, Conn.

Rickets

Discussion

Comparatively recently, general exposure to 1°E UVL was recognized as an important part of treatment. Since oral administration of vitamin D has been possible this pleasant treatment has almost disappeared. Late diagnosis or vitamin D resistant rickets may require surgical procedures to correct deformity, and therefore post-operative physiotherapy.

References to Section I

Chapter 4 (1)   Chapter 4 (3) (*b*)
Chapter 4 (3) (*a*)   Appendix 7

Further Reading:

Lloyd Roberts, G. C. (1971). *Orthopaedics in Infancy and Childhood.*
Ed. by J. Apley. London: Butterworths.
Sharrard, W. J. W. (1971). *Paediatric Orthopaedics and Fractures.*
Oxford and Edinburgh: Blackwell Scientific Publications.

Road traffic accidents

Discussion

Road traffic accidents produce an enormous variety of injuries.
The therapist may be involved in the respiratory care, or subsequently
as part of a neurological or orthopaedic rehabilitation programme.
Only general points will be discussed.

Respiration.   There may be direct trauma to the thoracic region
or depressed respiration due to general injuries. The patient may
require a tracheostomy. Physiotherapy should start immediately.
The aims and means are described in Section I.

Neurological.   Even if the patient is in coma, movements should
be started as soon as possible and the patient stimulated visually,
aurally and by touch. The authors have found that in the months of
recovery children sometimes remember events which took place
when they were considered to be deeply unconscious. So little is
known about the recovery process that we think it is essential that
the approach should be positive; no patient should ever be talked
over and around as though he were totally unaware.

Immediately after regaining consciousness there is often a
dramatic improvement and families may become euphoric as to the
eventual outcome. Almost inevitably a plateau is reached physically,
if not emotionally and intellectually. This fragmentation of recovery
makes rehabilitation particularly complicated. A long and comprehensive programme is required which may involve the teacher,
psychologist and psychiatrist as well as the medical and paramedical
professions.

Orthopaedic. Immediately following the accident physiotherapy will be included if appropriate.

During the recovery period a detailed functional assessment may be indicated to help the surgeon plan his treatment. Appropriate pre- and post-operative physiotherapy will be given.

From the moment of the accident, and overlapping all the areas discussed, the patient's posture must be carefully supervised. Unsuitable positions in bed may lead to unnecessary difficulties in rehabilitation.

References to Section I

Chapter 2	Chapter 4 (2) (*a*)	Appendix 3
Chapter 3 (Respiratory)	Appendix 1	Appendix 5
Chapter 4 (1)	Appendix 2	Appendix 6

Further Reading:

Brink, J. D., Garrett, A. L., Hale, W. R., Woo-Sam, J. and Nickel, V. L. (1970). 'Recovery of motor and intellectual function in children sustaining severe head injuries.' *Dev. Med. Child. Neurol.,* **12**, 565.

Rubella syndrome

Discussion

The severity of rubella syndrome varies considerably; visual difficulties and hearing loss together with mental retardation very often create the greatest disability. Bizarre hand and limb movements are frequently seen and mimic those more usually associated with other conditions. Some children also present with cerebral palsy. Physiotherapy will be part of management and its importance depends on the symptoms which each child presents.

References to Section I

Chapter 2	Appendix 1	Appendix 4
Chapter 4 (1)	Appendix 2	Appendix 6
Chapter 4 (2) (*a*)	Appendix 3	Appendix 8
Chapter 4 (2) (*b*)		

Scleroderma

Discussion

When this condition occurs in childhood there is a much greater possibility of regression than when it makes its first appearance in adult life. It is therefore essential to make every effort to prevent severe contractures occurring. Fingers and hands are most affected and physiotherapy is aimed at maintaining—or increasing—range of movement. Passive, assisted-active and active exercises must be given daily. If the condition of the skin allows, treatment in a pool is helpful.

References to Section I

Chapter 4 (1)   Appendix 8
Chapter 4 (2) (*d*)

Further Reading:

Duffield, M. H. (Ed.) (1969). *Exercises in Water*. London: Baillière, Tindall and Cassell.
Kiernander, B. (Ed.) (1965). *Physical Medicine in Paediatrics*. London: Butterworths.

Scoliosis

Discussion

It is outside the scope of this book to elaborate on the many varieties of scoliosis. From the point of view of physical treatment there are two significant groups: structural and postural.

Structural scoliosis has alteration of bone shape with rotation of vertebrae and the lateral curvature does not disappear on forward flexion. Examples are idiopathic scoliosis and congenital hemivertebra. Postural lateral curvature may have a structural cause, for example lower limb true shortening, but there is no vertebral rotation or significant structural change in the spine. Forward flexion eliminates the curve. Postural curves have many causes amongst which are: hemiplegia, preferred head turning in infants and thoracic surgery.

Physiotherapy may not be required because the condition is too mild or because the scoliosis is beyond physical treatment; in other cases physiotherapy has a limited part to play. The overall management depends on accurate diagnosis and long observation. Bracing and spinal fusion are often indicated. Specific exercises alone will not influence scoliosis, although general 'baby gymnastics' will help to prevent bad postural habits developing in suitably selected cases, particularly if other abnormalities are present.

Blount recommends an exercise programme combined with wearing a Milwaukee brace, which is frequently used for young children with a progressive curve. It is claimed that the incidence of success rises appreciably (Keim, 1972). Exercises are performed both in and out of the brace, practised at home, and then checked and supervised when the child attends a brace clinic. This is the system of treatment and supervision which the authors recommend.

Patients with a severe or progressive curve have a general displacement of mediastinal and abdominal viscera which leads, amongst other things, to a decrease in respiratory efficiency. Chest care is then an important part of treatment especially in disorders similar to muscular dystrophy. Respiratory care is also necessary if treatment is by corrective plasters or spinal fusion.

REFERENCE

Keim, H. A. (1972). 'Scoliosis': *Clinical Symposia CIBA* **24**, 1.

References to Section I

Further Reading:

Lloyd Roberts, G. C. (1971). *Orthopaedics in Infancy and Childhood.* Ed. by J. Apley. London: Butterworths.
Blount, W. P. and Bolinske, J. (1967). 'Physical therapy in the non-operative treatment of scoliosis.' *Phys. Ther.,* **47**, (10), 919.

Sinusitis

Discussion

It is many years since children with 'uncomplicated' sinusitis have been referred for physiotherapy. *See Cystic fibrosis* for sinusitis as a complication of polyps.

Spina bifida cystica

Discussion

The physiotherapy for this condition can be considered only with the other facets of treatment. The referring physician or surgeon should supervise a comprehensive treatment team.

References to Section I

Chapter 2	Chapter 4 (2) (*c*)	Appendix 3
Chapter 4 (1)	Appendix 1	Appendices 5–8

Further Reading:

Lloyd Roberts, G. C. (1971). *Orthopaedics in Infancy and Childhood.* Ed. by J. Apley. London: Butterworths.

Cane, F. R. (1969). 'Walking training of the young child with myelomeningocele.' *Physiotherapy*, **55**, (8), 322.

Holgate, L. (1970). *Physiotherapy for Spina Bifida Early Treatment.* Carshalton: Queen Mary's Hospital for Children.

Holgate, L. (1971). *Physiotherapy for Spina Bifida Further Management.* Carshalton: Queen Mary's Hospital for Children.

Nettles, O. (1972). *The Spina Bifida Baby.* Edinburgh: Scottish Spina Bifida Association.

Nettles, O. (1972). *Growing Up with Spina Bifida.* Edinburgh: Scottish Spina Bifida Association.

Edbrooke, H. (1970). 'The Royal Salop Infirmary "clicking splint".' *Physiotherapy*, **56**, (4), 148.

Martin, M. C. (1967). 'Spina bifida.' *Physiotherapy*, **53**, (9), 299.

Sharrard, W. J. W. (1971). *Paediatric Orthopaedics and Fractures.* Oxford and Edinburgh: Blackwell Scientific Publications.

Spina bifida occulta

Discussion

Many cases of spina bifida occulta present no symptoms. When they do occur the deformity most usually seen is pes cavus, and in more severe instances some degree of leg weakness. The patients may be referred to the physiotherapist for motor assessment and muscle testing. Physiotherapy will be needed following surgery.

References to Section I

Chapter 4 (1)   Chapter 4 (3) (*a*) (*b*)
Chapter 4 (2) (*d*) (*i*)

Further Reading:

Lloyd Roberts, G. C. (1971). *Orthopaedics in Infancy and Childhood.*
    Ed. by J. Apley. London: Butterworths.
Sharrard, W. J. W. (1971). *Paediatric Orthopaedics and Fractures.*
    Oxford and Edinburgh: Blackwell Scientific Publications.

Still's disease—juvenile rheumatoid arthritis

Discussion

There is some disagreement about the exact subgrouping of rheumatoid arthritis in childhood (Ansell and Bywaters, 1962). Initially, one joint only may be affected and no general systemic symptoms seen; or the child may have an acute fever with widespread joint tenderness. Whatever medical investigations and academic discussion are proceeding it is important that physiotherapy is included in the management of the patient as soon as any symptoms arise.

The primary aim of physiotherapy is to prevent deformity and the therapist should be in frequent contact with the physician.

Acute phase. A judicious mixture of rest and activity must be encouraged even if the child is febrile, and every effort made to avoid him being constantly in bed. Joints must be moved through as full a range as pain will allow every day and active movements encouraged. Splints are used to rest painful joints for restricted periods only, and nursing positions must be carefully supervised.

Hydrotherapy is important, and movements can often be encouraged and range increased in a pool long before it would otherwise be possible.

REFERENCE

Ansell, B. M. and Bywaters, E. G. L. (1962). 'Diagnosis of probable Still's disease and its outcome.' *Ann. Rheum. Dis.,* **21**, 253.

Sub-acute.   As the child's general condition improves his treatment needs to become more vigorous, and will be continued at home following discharge from hospital. Regular follow up at a hospital is essential.

Long-standing and quiescent condition.   Unfortunately an ideal treatment is not always possible for a variety of reasons. Deformity may already be present when the patient is first seen, or occur in spite of apparently adequate management. In these cases, serial splinting, manipulation, or surgery may be necessary. The emphasis will then be orthopaedic and physiotherapy management will be influenced by the surgical procedures undertaken.

References to Section I

Chapter 4 (1)   Chapter 4 (3) (*b*)   Appendix 8
Chapter 4 (3) (*a*)   Appendix 5

Further Reading:

Lloyd Roberts, G. C. (1971). *Orthopaedics in Infancy and Childhood.* Ed. by J. Apley. London: Butterworths.
Davis, B. C. (1967). 'A technique of re-education in the treatment pool.' *Physiotherapy*, **53**, (2), 57.
Duffield, M. H. (Ed.) (1969). *Exercises in Water*. London: Baillière, Tindall and Cassell.
Kiernander, B. (Ed.) (1965). *Physical Medicine in Paediatrics.* London: Butterworths.
Sharrard, W. J. W. (1971). *Paediatric Orthopaedics and Fractures.* Oxford and Edinburgh: Blackwell Scientific Publications.
Ansell, B. M. (1965). In *Clinical Rheumatology*. London: Churchill.

Talipes equino varus

Discussion

There are various methods of treating talipes equino varus, some of which do not include physiotherapy in infancy. We are used to a system of treatment which includes application of Robert Jones strapping and in this regime therapists are responsible for teaching the parents manipulations as well as for applying the strapping.

The programme continues from birth until the baby is about six months old (even if the hindfoot is released surgically at six to eight weeks) when he will start wearing Denis Browne hobble boots. Older children who have undergone recent surgery will require exercises and walking training. When dealing with the infant it is essential that the therapist is in close touch with the orthopaedic surgeon, and is informed of any additional congenital abnormalities.

References to Section I

Chapter 2	Chapter 4 (3) (*a*)	Chapter 4 (3) (*c*)
Chapter 4 (1)	Chapter 4 (3) (*b*)	Appendix 5

Further Reading:

Lloyd Roberts, G. C. (1971). *Orthopaedics in Infancy and Childhood.* Ed. by J. Apley. London: Butterworths.
Fripp, A. T. and Shaw, N. (1967). *Clubfoot.* Edinburgh: Livingstone.
Shaw, N. (1964). 'Comparison of three methods.' *Br. med. J.* **1**, 1084.
Sharrard, W. J. W. (1971). *Paediatric Orthopaedics and Fractures.* Oxford and Edinburgh: Blackwell Scientific Publications.

Torticollis

Discussion

Infants. The aim is to encourage active movement and prevent permanent muscle shortening. This is done by passive stretchings which must be instituted early, taught to the parents, and supervised frequently. The manipulations are difficult and can be distressing to perform; the parents need help to gain sufficient confidence. They should also be shown the best ways to hold and stimulate the baby so as to encourage as full a range of neck movements as possible. A brief birth history and reassurance that this is an isolated deformity is the only additional information needed by the physiotherapist.

Children. If the condition does not resolve and requires surgery this is usually planned to be done when the child is three or four years old. Stretchings into the corrected position must be given immediately post-operatively, and corrective postural exercises started. A Plastazote* collar is sometimes helpful. The initial post-

* Plastazote is a non-toxic foamed polyethylene with low flammability.

operative period is very trying for the patients. When the discomfort has subsided children are usually co-operative should they need to continue with exercises.

References to Section I

Chapter 2   Appendix 1
Chapter 4 (1)

Further Reading:

Lloyd Roberts, G. C. (1971). *Orthopaedics in Infancy and Childhood.* Ed. by J. Apley. London: Butterworths.
Sharrard, W. J. W. (1971). *Paediatric Orthopaedics and Fractures.* Oxford and Edinburgh: Blackwell Scientific Publications.

Trachea

See Congenital malformations

Ulcers

See Indolent ulcers

Upper respiratory tract infections

See Mouth breathers; Sinusitis

References to Section I

Chapter 2
Chapter 3

Viral infections

Discussion

The sequelae of viral infections may require physiotherapy, e.g. post-measles meningitis, vaccine encephalitis. These will then be treated as indicated.

Vitiligo

Discussion

This condition causes great distress to patient and family, especially when it occurs in dark-skinned races. No satisfactory remedy has been found, but the physiotherapist has a part to play in testing the efficiency of barrier creams to ultra-violet light, and occasionally in giving a course of UVL combined with orally administered drugs. Obviously a close liaison with the dermatologist is essential throughout any treatment.

Reference to Section I

Appendix 7

Further Reading:

Fischer, E. and Soloman, S. (1967). 'Physiologic effects of ultra-violet radiation.' In *Therapeutic Electricity and Ultra Violet Radiation*. Ed. by S. Licht, Elizabeth Licht, New Haven, Conn.

Werdnig Hoffmann's disease

Discussion

There is no known treatment for this condition and most children do not survive beyond five years of age. Nevertheless it is appropriate that physiotherapy should be part of the general management. Efforts should be made to prevent deformities occurring, and to encourage any possible active movement; although treatment is mostly directed to respiratory care.

Some cases do remit and there are a few adult survivors, all of whom are severely disabled. All children should receive treatment, not only as a short-term palliative, but in the positive hope that they will survive and that deformities and chronic respiratory disorder be prevented.

References to Section I

Chapter 2   Chapter 4 (1)   Appendix 6
Chapter 3   Appendix 5

Further Reading:

Lloyd Roberts, G. C. (1971). *Orthopaedics in Infancy and Childhood.* Ed. by J. Apley. London: Butterworths.

Kiernander, B. (Ed.) (1965). *Physical Medicine in Paediatrics.* London: Butterworths.

Further reading

Chapter 2

Bobath, B. and Finnie, N. R. (1970). 'Problems of communication between parents and staff in the treatment and management of children with cerebral palsy.' *Dev. Med. Child. Neurol.,* **12**, 629.

Chapter 3

Burton, L. (1972). 'An investigation into the problems occasioned for the child with cystic fibrosis.' In *Proceedings of 84th Annual General Meeting of I.C.A.A.*
Garbe, D. R. and McDonnell, H. *Lung Function Testing.* Vitalograph Ltd.
Groen, J. J. (1972). 'The mechanism of the disturbance of respiration during the asthmatic attack.' *Physiotherapy,* **58**, (11), 371.
McNicol, K. N. and Williams, H. B. (1973). 'Spectrum of asthma in children. 1: Clinical and physiological components.' *Br. med. J.* **4**, 7–11.
McNicol, K. N. and Williams, H. B. (1973). 'Spectrum of asthma in children. 2: Allergic components.' *Br. med. J.* **4**, 12–16.
McNicol, K. N., Williams, H. B., Allan, J. and McAndrew, I. (1973). 'Spectrum of asthma in children. 3: Psychological and social components.' *Br. med. J.* **4**, 16–20.
Morony, T. (1969). 'Cystic fibrosis.' *Austr. J. Phys.,* **XV**, (4), 125.
Rubin, S. (1967). 'Physiotherapy and cystic fibrosis.' *Physiotherapy,* **53**, (2), 51.
Young, W. F. (1967). 'Cystic fibrosis.' *Physiotherapy,* **53** (2), 48.

Chapter 4

Adams, R. C., Daniel, A. and Rullman, L. (1972). *Games, Sports and Exercises for the Physically Handicapped.* London: Heinemann.

Asher, D. (1974). *Postural Variations in Childhood*. London: Butterworths.

Bennett, R. L. (1952). 'Physical medicine in poliomyelitis—points of emphasis.' In *Poliomyelitis*, 261–269. Paper at 2nd International Poliomyelitis Conference, Lippincott.

Bleck, E. E. (1971). 'The shoeing of children: sham or science?' *Dev. Med. Child. Neurol., 13*, 188.

Blockley, J. and Miller, G. (1971). 'Feeding techniques with cerebral-palsied children.' *Physiotherapy, 57*, (7), 300.

Blount, W. P. and Bolinske, J. (1967). 'Physical therapy in the non-operative treatment of scoliosis.' *Phys. Ther., 47*, (10), 919.

Bobath, B. (1967). 'The very early treatment of cerebral palsy.' *Dev. Med. Child. Neurol., 9*, (4), 373.

Bobath, K. and Bobath, B. (1964). 'The facilitation of normal postural reactions and movements in the treatment of cerebral palsy.' *Physiotherapy, 50*, (8), 246.

Brink, J. D., Garrett, A. L., Hale, W. R., Woo-Sam, J. and Nickel, V. L. (1970). 'Recovery of motor and intellectual function in children sustaining severe head injuries.' *Dev. Med. Child. Neurol., 12*, 565.

Brunnstrom, S. (1956). *Methods Used to Elicit, Reinforce and Coordinate Muscular Response in Upper Motor Neuron Lesions. Am. Phys. Ther. Ass., O.V.R., Institute Papers*. New York: American Physical Therapy Association.

Campbell, E. D. R. and Green, E. A. (1970). 'Treatment of cerebral palsy in the severely subnormal.' *Rheum. Phys. Med. X*, 8.

Cane, F. R. (1969). 'Walking training of the young child with myelomeningocele.' *Physiotherapy, 55*, (8), 322.

Catto, A. M. and MacNaughton, A. (1966). 'Physiotherapy and occupational therapy in the management of the upper limb amputee.' *Physiotherapy, 52*, (6), 187.

Corner, B. (1968). 'Schooling for physically handicapped children—an introduction.' *Physiotherapy, 54*, (12), 434.

Cotton, E. (1970). 'Integration of treatment and education in cerebral palsy.' *Physiotherapy, 56*, (4), 143.

Cotton, E. (1965). 'The Institute of Movement Therapy and School for "Conductors" Budapest, Hungary.' *Dev. Med. Child. Neurol., 7*, 437.

Daniels, L., Williams, M. and Worthington, C. (1956). *Muscle Testing—Techniques of Manual Examination*. Philadelphia, Pa.: W. B. Saunders Co.

Dubowitz, V. (1968). 'The myopathies.' *Physiotherapy, 54*, (11), 384.

Edbrooke, H. (1970). 'The Royal Salop Infirmary "clicking splint".' *Physiotherapy,* **56**, (4), 148.

Field, A. (1968). 'Interdisciplinary work in a special school.' *Physiotherapy*, **54**, (12), 449.

Finnie, N. R. (1974). *Handling the Young Cerebral Palsied Child at Home. 2nd Ed.* London: Heinemann Medical Books.

Fripp, A. T. and Shaw, N. (1967). *Clubfoot.* Edinburgh: Livingstone.

Gardiner, M. D. (1963). *The Principles of Exercise Therapy.* London: G. Bell.

Goff, B. (1969). 'Appropriate afferent stimulation.' *Physiotherapy*, **55**, (1), 9.

Gray, E. R. (1969). 'The role of leg muscles in variations of the arches in normal and flat feet.' *Phys. Ther.,* **49**, 10, 1084.

Halpern, D., Kottke, F. J., Burrill, C., Fiterman, C., Popp, J. and Palmer, S. (1970). 'Training of control of head posture in children with cerebral palsy.' *Dev. Med. Child. Neurol.,* **12**, 290.

Holgate, L. (1970). *Physiotherapy for Spina Bifida Early Treatment.* Carshalton: Queen Mary's Hospital for Children.

Holgate, L. (1971). *Physiotherapy for Spina Bifida Further Management.* Carshalton: Queen Mary's Hospital for Children.

Holt, K. S. (1965). *Assessment of Cerebral Palsy.* **1**. London: Lloyd-Luke (Medical Books).

Holt, K. S. and Reynell, J. K. (1967). *Assessment of Cerebral Palsy.* **2**. London: Lloyd-Luke (Medical Books).

Huckstep, R. L. (1970). 'Poliomyelitis in Uganda.' *Physiotherapy*, **56**, (8), 347.

Hughes, N. A. S. (1971). 'Developmental physiotherapy for mentally handicapped babies.' *Physiotherapy*, **57**, (9), 399.

Illingworth, R. S. (1966). *The Development of the Infant and Young Child, Normal and Abnormal.* Edinburgh and London: Livingstone.

Kettlewell, B. (1956). 'The unique effect of fatigue in poliomyelitis.' *Physiotherapy*, **42**, (2), 45.

Knott, M. and Voss, D. E. (1968). *Proprioceptive neuro-muscular facilitation.* New York: Harper Row.

Licht, S. (Ed.). (1958). *Therapeutic Exercises.* Elizabeth Licht, New Haven, Conn.

Lloyd Roberts, G. C. (1971). *Orthopaedics in Infancy and Childhood.* Ed. by J. Apley. London: Butterworths.

Lovell, L. M. (1973). 'The Yeovil opportunity group: A play group for multiple handicapped children.' *Physiotherapy*, **59**, (8), 251.

Martin, J. P. (1965). 'Tilting reactions and disorders of the basal ganglia.' *Brain*, **88**, 855.

Martin, M. C. (1967). 'Spina bifida.' *Physiotherapy*, **53**, (9), 299.

Morton, J. and Malins, P. (1971). 'The correction of spinal deformities by halo-pelvic traction.' *Physiotherapy*, **57**, (12), 576.

Nettles, O. (1972). *The Spina Bifida Baby*. Edinburgh: Scottish Spina Bifida Association.

Nettles, O. (1972). *Growing Up with Spina Bifida*. Edinburgh: Scottish Spina Bifida Association.

Pearson, F. A. and Spiers, B. W. (1966). 'Teamwork in the management of dysmelic children.' *Physiotherapy*, **52**, (6), 197.

Peterkin, H. W. (1969). 'The neuromuscular system and the reeducation of movement.' *Physiotherapy*, **55**, (4), 145.

Pohl, J. F. and Kenny, E. (1943). *The Kenny Concept of Infantile Paralysis and its Treatment*. St. Paul: Bruce.

Reynolds, R. J. S. (1956). *Physical Measures in the Treatment of Poliomyelitis*. London: Faber and Faber.

Robson, P. (1970). 'Shuffling, hitching, scooting or sliding: some observations in 30 otherwise normal children.' *Dev. Med. Child. Neurol.*, **12**, 608.

Rood, M. (1967). 'Miss Rood's approach.' *Am. J. phys. Med.*, **46**, 1.

Sharrard, W. J. W. (1967). *Paralysis, Upper and Lower Motor Neuron: Clinical Surgery.*, **13**, Orthopaedics London: Butterworths.

Sharrard, W. J. W. (1971). *Paediatric Orthopaedics and Fractures*. Oxford and Edinburgh: Blackwell Scientific Publications.

Shaw, N. (1964). 'Comparison of three methods.' *Br. med. J.* **1**, 1084.

Stamp, W. G. (1962). 'Bracing in cerebral palsy.' *J. Bone Jt. Surg.*, **44A**, 1457.

Walton, J. N. (1956). 'Benign congenital hypotonia.' *Lancet* **1**, 1023.

Appendix 1

'An Exploratory and Analytical Survey of Therapeutic Exercise.' (1966). North West Univ: Special Therapeutic Exercise Project. *Am. J. Phys. Med.*, **46**, (1), 1967.

Bobath, K. and Bobath, B. (1964). 'The facilitation of normal postural reactions and movements in the treatment of cerebral palsy.' *Physiotherapy*, **50**, (8), 246.

Halpern, D., Kottke, F. J., Burrill, C., Fiterman, C., Popp, J. and Palmer, S. (1970). 'Training of control of head posture in children with cerebral palsy.' *Dev. Med. Child. Neurol.*, **12**, 290.

Horton, M. E. (1971). 'The development of movement in young children.' *Physiotherapy*, **57**, (4), 149.

Hughes, N. A. S. (1971). 'Developmental physiotherapy for mentally handicapped babies.' *Physiotherapy*, **57**, (9), 399.

Knott, M. and Voss, D. E. (1968). *Proprioceptive neuro-muscular facilitation*. New York: Harper Row.

Peterkin, H. W. (1969). 'The neuromuscular system and the re-education of movement.' *Physiotherapy*, **55**, (4), 145.

Appendix 2

Bobath, B. (1971). *Abnormal Postural Reflex Activity Caused by Brain Lesions*. London: Heinemann.

Bobath, K. and Bobath, B. (1964). 'The facilitation of normal postural reactions and movements in the treatment of cerebral palsy.' *Physiotherapy*, **50**, (8), 246.

Appendix 3

Bobath, K. and Bobath, B. (1964). 'The facilitation of normal postural reactions and movements in the treatment of cerebral palsy.' *Physiotherapy*, **50**, (8), 246.

Milani-Comparetti, A. and Gidoni, E. A. (1967). 'Routine developmental examination in normal and retarded children.' *Dev. Med. Child. Neurol.*, **9**, 631.

Appendix 5

Brooks, M. B. (1969). 'Success and failure in infant prosthetic fitting.' *Rehabilitation*, **70**, 31.

Day, B. H. (1972). *Orthopaedic Appliances*. London: Faber and Faber.

Edbrooke, H. (1970). 'The Royal Salop Infirmary "clicking splint".' *Physiotherapy*, **56**, (4), 148.

Kennedy, J. M. (1974). *Orthopaedic splints and appliances*. London: Ballière Tindall.

Morton, J. and Malins, P. (1971). 'The correction of spinal deformities by halo-pelvic traction.' *Physiotherapy*, **57**, (12), 576.

Nangle, E. J. (1951). *Instruments and Apparatus in Orthopaedic Surgery*. Oxford: Blackwell Scientific Publications.

Stamp, W. G. (1962). 'Bracing in cerebral palsy.' *J. Bone Jt. Surg.*, **44A**, 1457.

Von Werssowetz, O. (1962). 'Basic principles of lower extremity bracing.' *Am. J. phys. Med.*, **41**, 156.

Appendix 7

Bauwens, P. (1963). 'New ways with a venerable remedy.' *Physiotherapy*, **49**, (2), 40.

Dyson, M. and Pond, J. B. (1970). 'The effect of pulsed ultrasound on tissue regeneration.' *Physiotherapy*, **56**, (4), 136.

Dyson, M. and Pond, J. B. (1973). 'The effects of ultrasound on circulation.' *Physiotherapy*, **59**, (9), 284.

Fischer, E. and Soloman, S. (1967). 'Physiologic effects of ultraviolet radiation.' In *Therapeutic Electricity and Ultra Violet Radiation*. Ed. by S. Licht, Elizabeth Licht, New Haven, Conn.

Harvey, B. R. and Elphick, A. M. (1969). 'Electrotherapy.' *Physiotherapy*, **55**, (5), 198.

Lehmann, J. F. (1965). 'Ultrasound therapy.' In *Therapeutic Heat and Cold*. Ed. by S. Licht, Elizabeth Licht, New Haven, Conn.

Licht, S. (Ed.) (1965). *Therapeutic Heat and Cold*. Elizabeth Licht, New Haven, Conn.

Licht, S. (Ed.) (1967). *Therapeutic Electricity and Ultra Violet Radiation*. Elizabeth Licht, New Haven, Conn.

Patrick, M. K. (1973). 'Ultrasonic therapy—has it a place in the 70's?' *Physiotherapy*, **59**, (9), 282.

Russell, J. G. B. and Jones, V. P. (1973). 'The uses and possible hazards of diagnostic ultrasound in medicine.' *Physiotherapy*, **59**, (9), 279.

Stephens, W. G. S. (1973). 'The assessment of muscle denervation by electrical stimulation.' *Physiotherapy*, **59**, (9), 292.

Stillwell, G. K. (1965). 'General principles of thermotherapy.' In *Therapeutic Heat and Cold*. Ed. by S. Licht, Elizabeth Licht, New Haven, Conn.

Summer, W. and Patrick, M. K. (1964). *Ultrasonic Therapy*. Amsterdam: Elsevier.

Von Werssowetz, O. D. (1965). 'Heat in neuromuscular disorders.' In *Therapeutic Heat and Cold*. Ed. by S. Licht, Elizabeth Licht, New Haven, Conn.

Williams, N. E. and Yates, D. A. H. (1973). 'Electrodiagnosis and electromyography.' *Physiotherapy*, **59**, (9), 288.

Willie, C. D. (1969). 'Interferential therapy.' *Physiotherapy*, **55**, (12), 503.

Appendix 8

Davis, B. C. (1967). 'A technique of re-education in the treatment pool.' *Physiotherapy*, **53**, (2), 57.
Duffield, M. H. (Ed.) (1969). *Exercises in Water*. London: Baillière, Tindall and Cassell.

Appendix 9

Glick, G. N. and Lucas, M. (1969). 'Ice therapy.' *Ann. Phys. Med.*, **10**, 70.
Haines, J. (1967). 'A survey of recent development in cold therapy.' *Physiotherapy*, **53**, (7), 222.
Licht, S. (1965). 'Local cryotherapy.' In *Therapeutic Heat and Cold*. Ed. by S. Licht, Elizabeth Licht, New Haven, Conn.
McGowan, H. L. (1967). 'Effects of cold application on maximal isometric contraction.' *Phys. Ther.*, **47**, (3), 185.
Marshall, R. S. (1971). 'Cold therapy in the treatment of pressure sores.' *Physiotherapy*, **57**, (8), 372.

General

Ansell, B. M. (1965). In *Clinical Rheumatology*. London: Churchill.
Burnett, C. M. and Johnson, E. W. (1971). 'The development of gait in childhood.' *Dev. Med. Child. Neurol.*, **13**, (2), 196.
Greg, G. (1964). 'The haemophiliac joint and its treatment by physical methods.' *Physiotherapy*, **50**, (12), 394.
Illingworth, R. S. (1968). 'How to help a child achieve his best.' *J. Pediat.*, **73**, 61.
Kiernander, B. (Ed.) (1965). *Physical Medicine in Paediatrics*. London: Butterworths.
Murray, M. P., Drought, A. B. and Kory, R. C. (1964). 'Walking patterns of normal men.' *J. Bone Jt. Surg.*, **46A**, (2), 335.
Murray, M. P. (1967). 'Patterns of sagittal rotation of the upper limbs in walking.' *Phys. Ther.*, **47**, (4), 272.
Perry, J. (1967). 'The mechanics of walking. A clinical interpretation.' *J. Am. phys. ther. Ass.*, **47**, (9), 778.

Scrutton, D. R. (1969). 'Footprint sequences of normal children under five years old.' *Dev. Med. Child. Neurol.*, **11**, 44.

Spiers, B. (1968). 'Physiotherapy in a hospital special school.' *Physiotherapy*, **54**, (12), 452.

Trussell, E. C. and Hayne, J. C. R. (1970). 'Physiotherapy in the treatment of burns and plastic surgery.' *Physiotherapy*, **56**, (3), 150.

Index